Oral and Maxillofacial Surgery

Oral and Maxillofacial Surgery

Editor: Gideon Schmidt

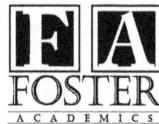

FA
FOSTER
ACADEMICS

www.fosteracademics.com

www.fosteracademics.com

FA
FOSTER
ACADEMICS

Cataloging-in-Publication Data

Oral and maxillofacial surgery / edited by Gideon Schmidt.
    p. cm.
Includes bibliographical references and index.
ISBN 978-1-63242-819-6
1. Face--Surgery. 2. Mouth--Surgery. 3. Maxilla--Surgery. I. Schmidt, Gideon.
RD523 .O73 2019
617.520 59--dc23

Foster Academics,
118-35 Queens Blvd., Suite 400,
Forest Hills, NY 11375, USA

ISBN 978-1-63242-819-6 (Hardback)

Contents

Preface

The surgical specialty concerned with the treatment of several disorders and defects in the face, head, neck, jaws, and the hard and soft tissues of the oral and maxillofacial region is known as oral and maxillofacial surgery. It is considered to be an important sub-speciality of dentistry. A medical practitioner who has specialized in the treatment of the entire craniomaxillofacial complex, which consists of the anatomical area of the mouth, skull, jaws, and face, is called an oral and maxillofacial surgeon. Some of the surgical procedures performed under this field include dentoalveolar surgery, genioplasty, orthognathic surgery, rhinoplasty, otoplasty, oculoplastics and septoplasty, among many others. This book is compiled in such a manner, that it will provide in-depth knowledge about the theory and practice of oral and maxillofacial surgery. It brings forth some of the most innovative concepts and elucidates the unexplored aspects of oral and maxillofacial surgery. The book is appropriate for students seeking detailed information in this area as well as for doctors and experts.

This book has been the outcome of endless efforts put in by authors and researchers on various issues and topics within the field. The book is a comprehensive collection of significant researches that are addressed in a variety of chapters. It will surely enhance the knowledge of the field among readers across the globe.

It gives us an immense pleasure to thank our researchers and authors for their efforts to submit their piece of writing before the deadlines. Finally in the end, I would like to thank my family and colleagues who have been a great source of inspiration and support.

Editor

Guided Bone Regeneration Technique Using Hyaluronic Acid in Oral Implantology

Fatih Özan, Metin Şençimen, Aydın Gülses and
Mustafa Ayna

Abstract

Guided bone regeneration is a term used to describe the use of the barrier membranes to enhance complete osteogenesis by preventing the rapid ingrowth of fibroblasts into a bony defect and promoting the migration of osteogenic cells from adjacent bony edges or bone marrow into the defect in an unimpeded fashion. Hyaluronic acid (HA) is a glycosaminoglycan of the general formula $(C14H22NO11)n$ and is an essential component of the extracellular matrix in connective tissue, which is found in abundance in the alveolar environment. The most important function of HA is its involvement in tissue healing and repair. It has been shown that HA stimulates cell proliferation, migration and angiogenesis, re-epithelialization and proliferation of basal keratinocytes and reduces collagen and scar tissue formation. This text presents our clinical experiences and outcomes following HA applications in various implant surgery procedures. According to our clinical outcomes, HA is a highly promising material for improving therapeutic outcomes for oral implantology.

Keywords: guided bone regeneration, hyaluronic acid, oral implantology, bone reconstruction, advanced oral surgery

1. Introduction

Loss of alveolar bone can result in secondary to periodontal diseases, periapical pathologies, maxillary sinus pneumatization or trauma to teeth and adjacent structures. Damage of the osseous structures during tooth extraction procedures may also result in bone loss of various types and severity. Sufficient alveolar bone volume and favorable architecture of the alveolar ridge are essential to obtain ideal functional and esthetic prosthetic reconstruction following implant therapy [1]. In order to overcome the problems related to osseous defects adjacent to implants and/or implant recipient sites, Dahlin and colleagues spearheaded early research on guided bone regeneration (GBR) techniques [2–4]. Herein, we present the technique.

2. Guided bone regeneration

GBR is a term used to describe the use of barrier membranes to enhance complete osteogenesis by preventing the rapid ingrowth of fibroblasts into a bony defect and promoting the migration of osteogenic cells from the adjacent bony edges or bone marrow into the defect in an unimpeded fashion [5]. Nowadays, various types of dental GBR materials have been developed, which can be grouped together as either non-resorbable or resorbable membranes.

3. Non-resorbable membranes

The first and recently mostly used commercial membrane was produced from Teflon® (e-PTFE). According to the results of various studies focusing on the efficacy of e-PTFE, predictable outcomes were observed, especially in ridge augmentation using it either alone or in combination with osseous grafting. However, membrane exposure, which permits a communication between the oral environment and newly forming tissues, increasing the potential for infection and decreasing the likelihood of regeneration, has been a frequent post-surgical complication associated with the use of non-resorbable membranes [6]. Moreover, non-resorbable membranes must be retrieved by employing a second surgical procedure [7].

4. Resorbable membranes

There are mainly three types of biologically resorbable membranes: (1) polyglycoside synthetic copolymers, (2) collagen and (3) calcium sulfate.

Collagen is the principal component of connective tissue and provides structural support for them. Collagen membranes are the most widely used resorbable membranes in implant surgery. They have various advantages such as hemostasis, chemotaxis, biotolerability, bioresorbtion, slow absorbtion and ease of manipulation compared to e-PTFE.

Hyaluronic acid (HA) is a glycosaminoglycan with a chemical formula $(C14H22NO11)n$ **and also found in abundance in the connective tissues of maxillary and mandibular tooth bearing areas** [8]. HA is particularly dense in the superficial layers of the buccal mucosa where it contributes to the epithelial barrier effect, at the same time enhancing both the stability and the elasticity of the peripheral connective tissue.

The most important function of HA is its involvement in tissue healing and repair [9, 10]. In the literature, it has been shown that HA stimulates cell proliferation, migration and angiogenesis, re-epithelialization and proliferation of basal keratinocytes and reduces collagen and scar tissue formation [11, 12].

In covalently cross-linked condition, HA forms a hydrophilic polymer network which may absorb its dry weight in water a multiple of times [13]. This lubricious property combined with its biocompatibility has led to different medical applications of HA in dermatology, ophthalmology, orthopedics, plastic surgery, and more recently, implantology, in order to benefit from its properties against inflammation and infection together with its capacity to promote wound healing.

Owing to that, HA is used as an effective medication for treatment of recurrent aphthous ulcers [14], as an adjuvant treatment for gingivitis [15], to enhance healing of tooth extraction socket [16] and interdental papillae reconstruction [17]. More recently, cross-linked HA products were used as gel barriers to cover the osseous defects around the implants and implant recipient sites and thereby promoting GBR. Claar performed a lateral coverage of the augmentation followed by use of cross-linked HA in gel form, which was developed especially for GBR [18].

The principles of GBR applications are as follows [19, 20]:

Cell exclusion: Crating a barrier to prevent forming fibrous connective tissue by epithelial cells.

Tenting: New wound space beneath the membrane must be regenerated solely from around soft tissues so that high quality of new tissue can be gained.

Scaffolding: At first, a fibrin clot is seen in this space which is a scaffold for progenitor cells. Adjacent hard tissues serve as a storage for stem cells.

Stabilization: To gain successful healing, the defective area must be protected from environmental effects such as flap movement, bacterial invasion, exposure of region, etc. by fixing the membrane into position.

It is well known that HA is a biodegradable, biocompatible, non-toxic, non-immunogenic and non-inflammatory linear polysaccharide. These properties demonstrate the superiority of HA by providing high biocompatibility and tissue integrity as a barrier membrane.

As mentioned above, the placement and stabilization of the membrane play a key role in the success of GBR. Therefore, the surgeon's skill and experience are of great importance. In addition, the need for removal of the mini bone screws placed for the stabilization of the membrane during implant insertion surgery necessitates a larger flap design and excessive exposure of the surgical field, especially in lateral sinus elevation procedures. Claar [18] has also proclaimed that, because of its high viscosity, HA is readily applicable and has high positional stability.

Marinucci *et al.* [21] evaluated the effects of bioabsorbable and non-resorbable membranes on human osteoblast activity *in vitro.* Human osteoblasts were cultured on bioabsorbable membranes made of collagen, HA, and poly DL-lactide, and e-PTFE. The results showed that collagen and HA increased secretion of TGF-β1, a growth factor involved in bone remodeling. It may be concluded that bioabsorbable membranes, particularly collagen and HA, can promote bone regeneration through their effects on osteoblasts. Besides that, HA and bioabsorbable membranes significantly increased collagen synthesis and alkaline phosphatase activity.

Membranes must remain in place until cells capable of regeneration are established at the wound site. Blumenthal [22] showed that collagen membranes cross-linked with formaldehyde can last 6 to 8 weeks before being absorbed, whereas non-cross-linked membranes lose their structural integrity in 7 days. HA gel in cross-linked form can last up to 3–4 weeks in the surgical field, which could be accepted as an appropriate term for enhancement of osteopromotion. HA is a highly promising material for improving therapeutic outcomes in dental implantology.

The aim of this section is to present clinical outcomes following HA applications in different implant surgery procedures.

5. Technique

5.1. Bone defects around dental implants

A 43-year-old healthy male patient admitted to our department due to the loss of his upper left lateral incisor was assessed. According to his history, the tooth was extracted 4 months ago following an unsuccessful endodontic treatment. A computerized tomography revealed the presence of a bone defect located adjacent to the missing tooth (**Figure 1**).

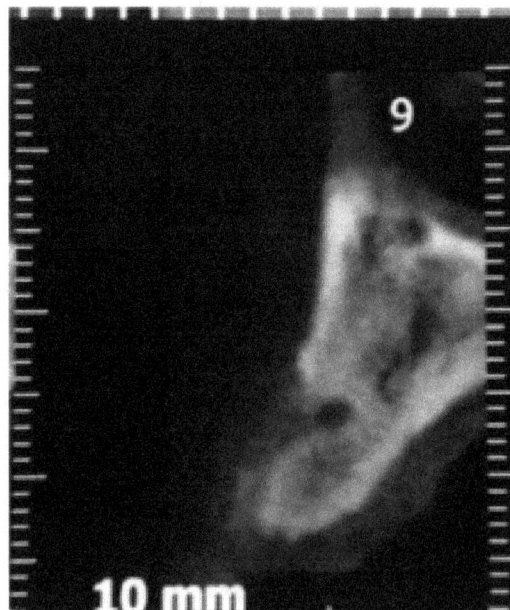

Figure 1. A computerized tomography scan revealed the presence of a bone defect located adjacent to the missing tooth.

After consultations with the prosthodontist, it was decided to insert an implant into the corresponding area. Under local anesthesia, a full thickness flap was raised and the bone defect and the implant recipient site were exposed. The granulation tissue were thoroughly curetted and the defect became more apparent (**Figure 2**).

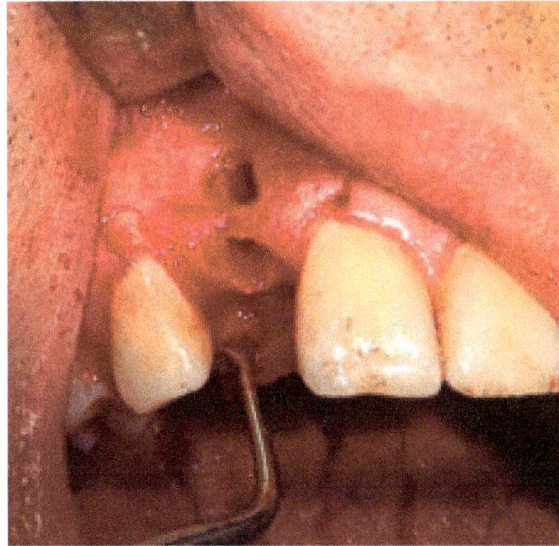

Figure 2. The remaining granulation tissues were thoroughly curetted and the defect became more apparent.

The implant site was prepared. A 3.4 × 11 mm implant (Bone Trust, Medical Instinct Zahn Implantate, Bovenden, Germany) was placed (**Figure 3**).

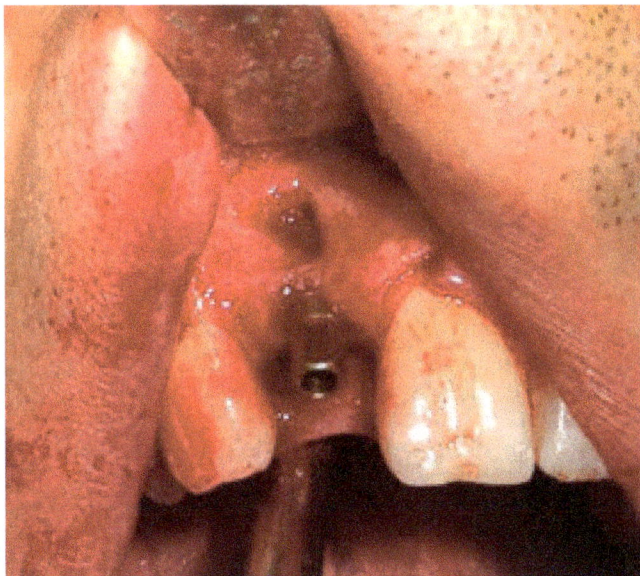

Figure 3. Placement of the implant.

The defect was grafted by using bioactive glass material (Leonardo, Naturelize, Hirschberg, Germany) mixed with non-cross-linked HA (Tissue Support Hyaluronic Acid Liquid Gel, Hyadent Bioscience GmbH, Ransbach-Baumbach, Germany) (**Figure 4**).

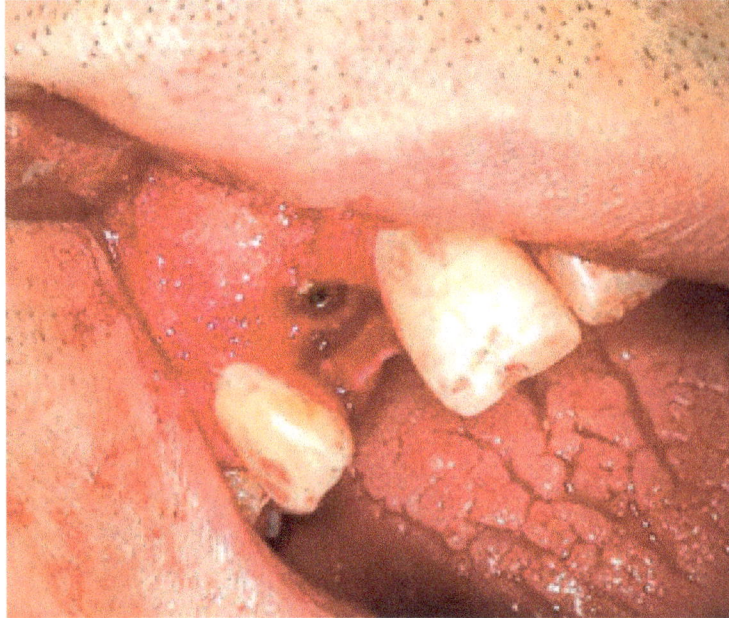

Figure 4. The defect was grafted by using bioactive glass material mixed with non-cross-linked HA.

The surgical field was covered by using cross-linked HA gel to avoid epithelial ingrowth to the grafted area. After closure of the surgical field with 4/0 silk sutures, the remaining cross-linked HA gel (Flex Barrier Hyaluronic Acid Gel, Hyadent Bioscience Gmbh, Ransbach-Baumbach, Germany) was injected into the surgical field in order to obtain a more predictable soft tissue profile and benefit from antibacterial properties of the material (**Figure 5**).

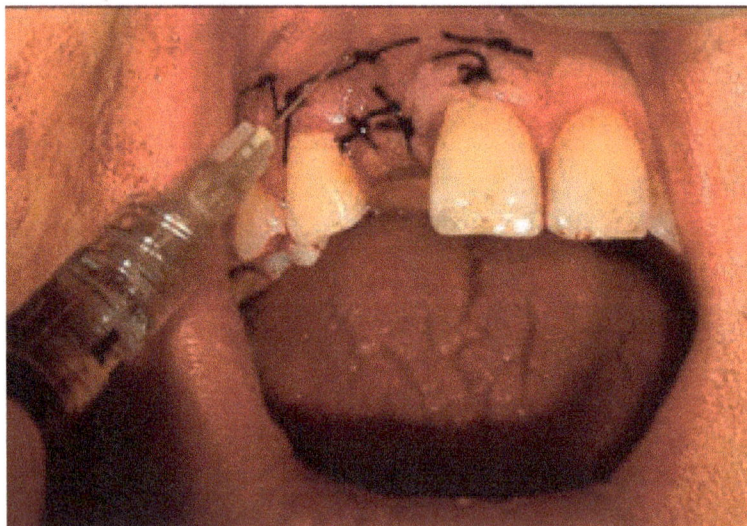

Figure 5. The injection of the remaining cross-linked HA into the surgical field.

Four months after implant placement (**Figure 6**), an ideal implant-bone contact was observed and the implant was functionally loaded. The patient was functionally and esthetically satisfied.

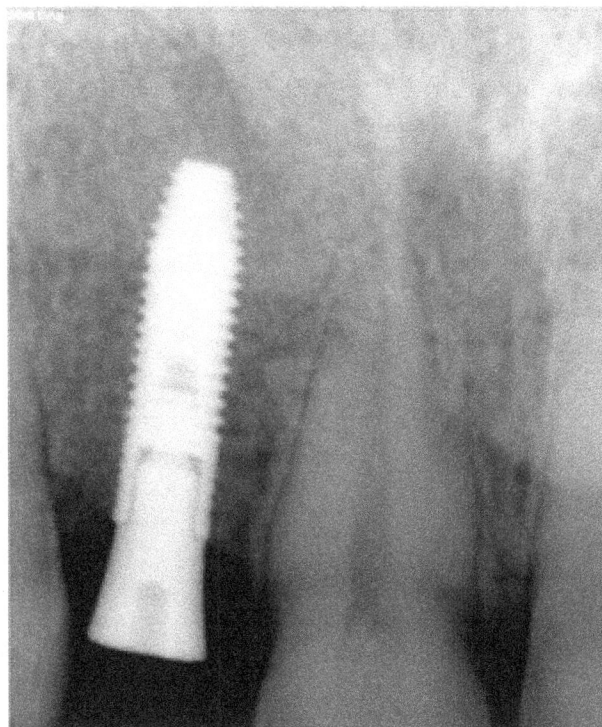

Figure 6. Four months after implant placement, an ideal implant-bone contact was observed.

5.2. Immediate post-extraction implant placement

A 34-year-old healthy female patient was admitted following the fracture of her upper left second premolar. On the clinical and radiographical examination, it was observed that upper left first and second premolars were unrestorable (**Figure 7**).

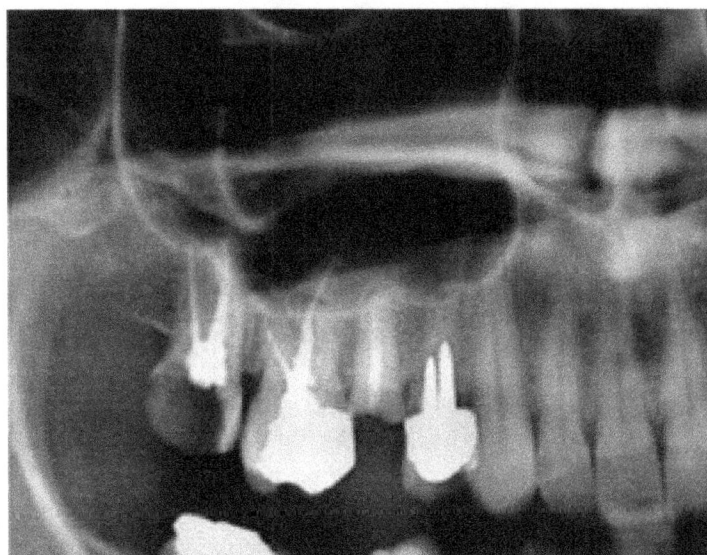

Figure 7. Radiological view of the upper right quadrant.

After consultation with the department of prosthodontics, it was decided to extract both teeth and to place implants simultaneously. Under local anesthesia, a full thickness flap was raised, both teeth were extracted (**Figure 8**) and two 5 × 11 mm Bone Trust implants (Bone Trust, Medical Instinct Zahn Implantate, Bovenden, Germany) were placed (**Figure 9**).

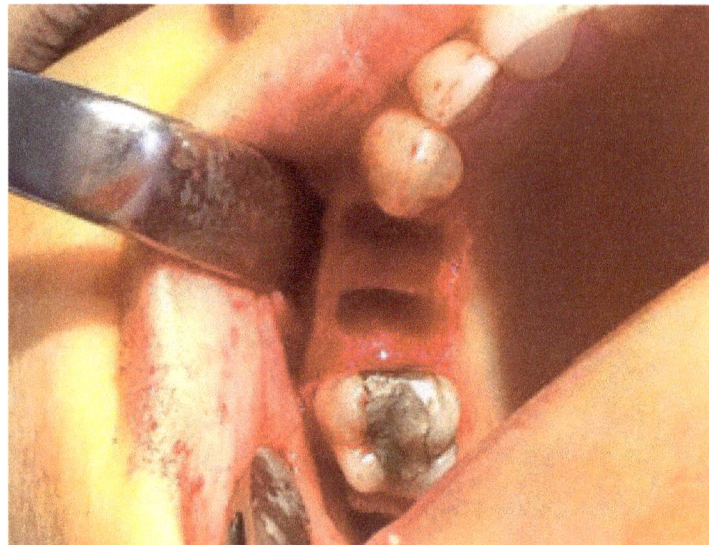

Figure 8. Intra-oral view after extraction of the upper first and second premolars.

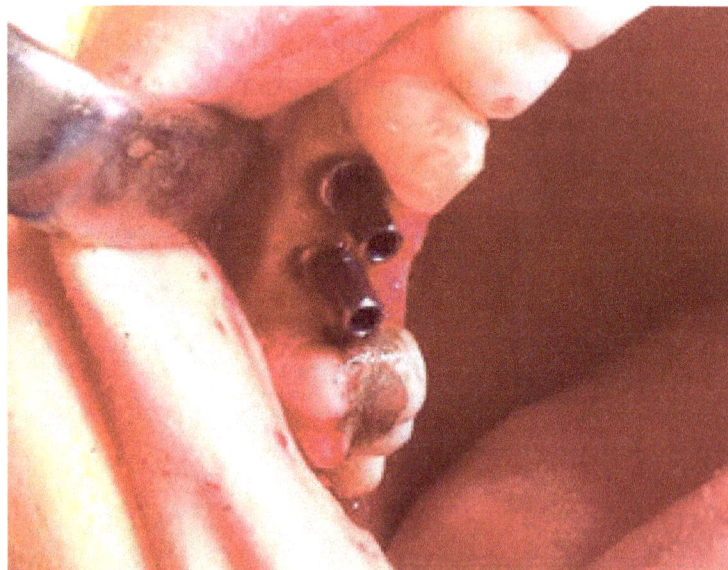

Figure 9. Placement of the implants. Please note the gap between the implants and the alveolus.

A gap was observed between the implant and the extraction socket, and these defects were grafted by using bioactive glass material (Leonardo, Naturelize, Hirschberg, Germany) mixed with non-cross-linked HA gel (Tissue Support Hyaluronic Acid Liqui Gel, Hyadent Bioscience Gmbh, Ransbach-Baumbach, Germany) (**Figure 10**).

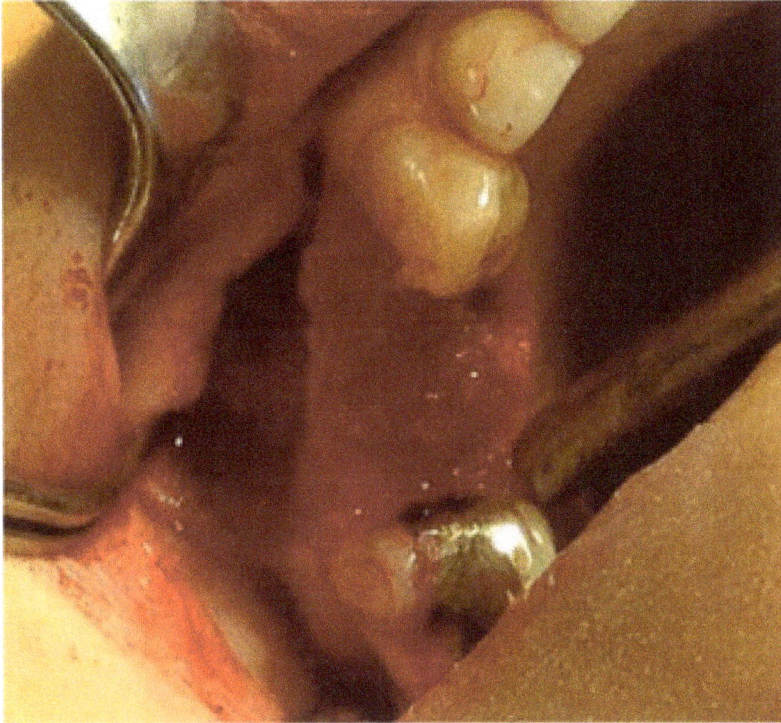

Figure 10. Grafting of the area with bioactive glass material mixed with non-cross-linked HA.

A cross-linked HA gel (Flex Barrier Hyaluronic Acid Gel, Hyadent Bioscience Gmbh, Ransbach-Baumbach, Germany) was injected over the implants and the graft material. Three months after implant placement (**Figure 11**), the implant was functionally loaded. The patient was satisfied both esthetically and functionally (**Figure 12**).

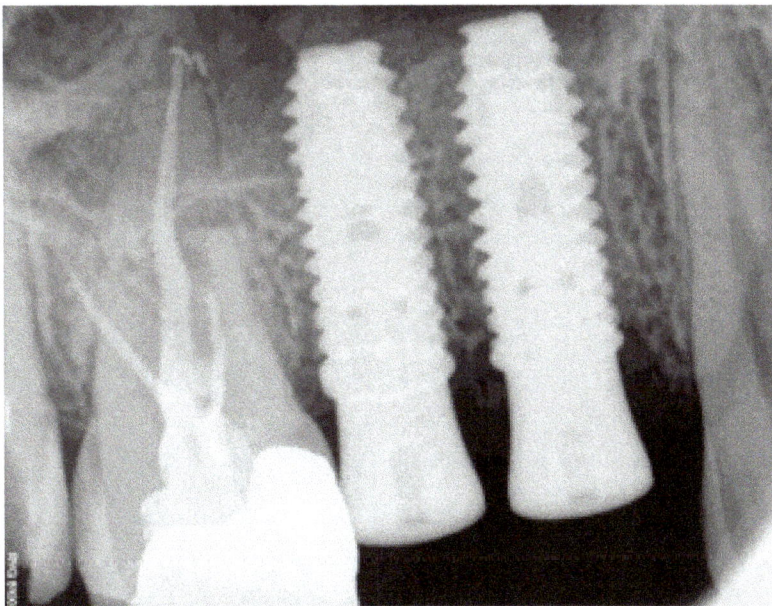

Figure 11. Three months after implant placement, an ideal implant-bone contact was observed.

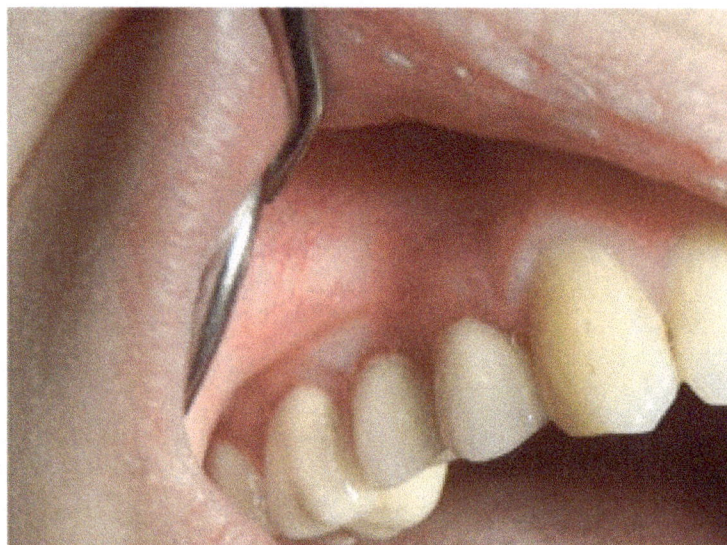

Figure 12. Clinical view after prosthetic procedure.

5.3. Sinus bone grafting

A 44-year-old healthy female patient presented to our department and requested a fixed prosthesis of the right maxillary posterior region. The teeth had to be removed at another clinic as a result of failed endodontic procedures. Clinical and radiological examinations showed the lack of an adequate vertical bone, but sufficient width of the alveolar ridge. Given that the residual vertical bone height was ≤3 mm (**Figure 13**), we planned to insert the implants following the sinus floor augmentation procedure.

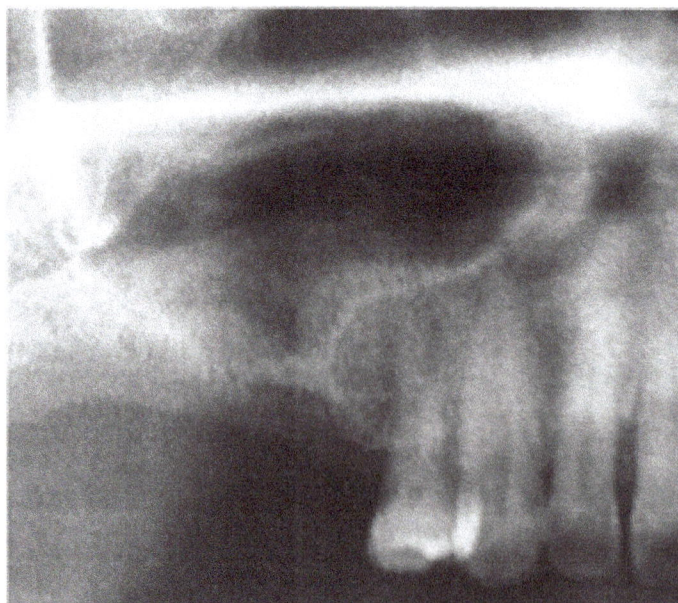

Figure 13. Preoperative radiological view.

A trapezoid incision was made under local anesthesia to reflect a mucoperiosteal flap. The vestibular portion of the maxillary sinus was exposed, a maxillary sinus window was prepared and the sinus membrane was elevated. The sinus cavity was augmented with a bioactive glass bone graft material (Leonardo, Naturelize, Hirschberg, Germany), which we had mixed with non-cross-linked HA (Tissue Support Hyaluronic Acid Liqui Gel, Hyadent Bioscience Gmbh, Ransbach-Baumbach, Germany) extra-orally (**Figure 14**), and the lateral coverage of the augmentation site was made by using cross-linked HA gel (Flex Barrier Hyaluronic Acid Gel, Hyadent Bioscience Gmbh, Ransbach-Baumbach, Germany) (**Figure 15**).

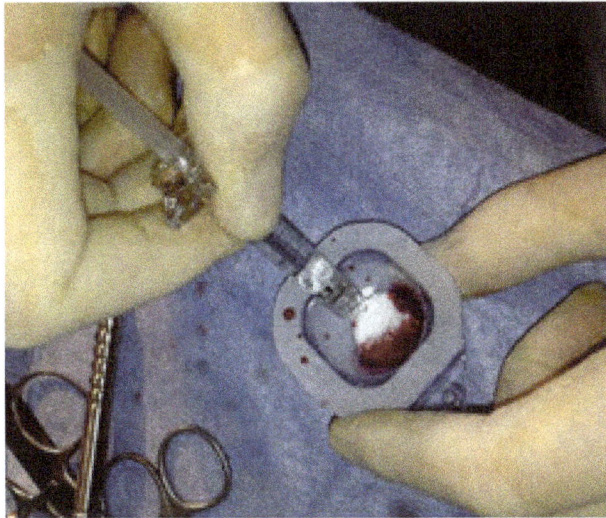

Figure 14. Mixing procedure of the bioactive glass bone graft material with non-cross-linked HA.

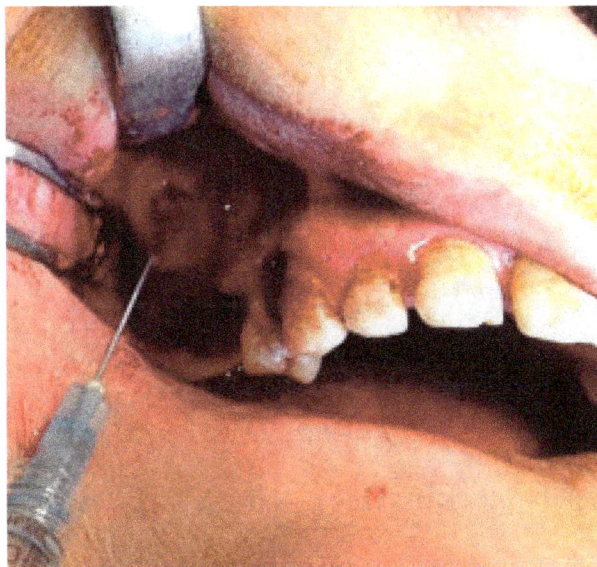

Figure 15. Augmentation of the sinus cavity with bioactive glass material mixed with non-cross-linked HA. Lateral coverage of the augmentation site was made by using cross-linked HA gel.

On radiographic examination 5 months postoperatively, particulated structure of the graft material was not seen and radio-opaque structure resembling the newly formed bone was observed (**Figure 16**).

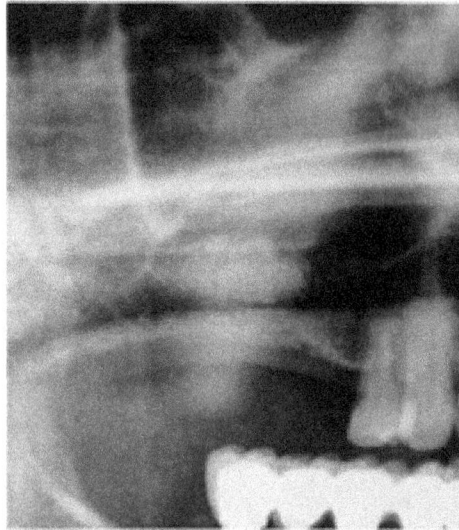

Figure 16. On the radiographic examination 5 months postoperatively, radio-opaque structure resembling the newly formed bone was observed.

Two implants (Oxy Biomec SRL, Colico, Italy) of 4, 5 × 10 mm were placed (**Figure 17**).

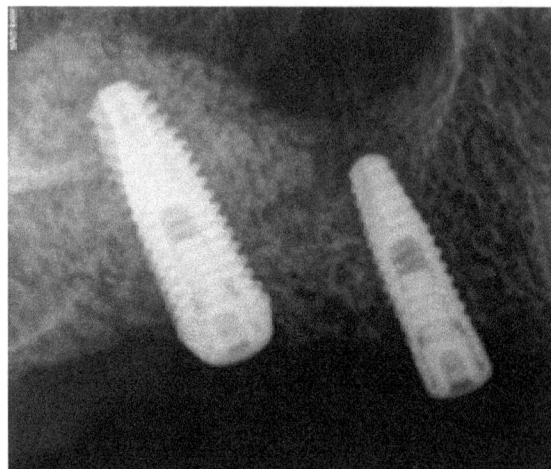

Figure 17. Placement of the implants.

The implants were surgically exposed and the prosthetic procedures were performed.

5.4. Covering of the autologous bone graft recipient sites (as a barrier membrane)

A 54-year-old female patient was admitted due to the difficulties in eating secondary to edentulousim of her lower left posterior mandible. According to her medical history, she was under steroid therapy due to lupus erythematosus. Clinically and radiographically, the corresponding area was extremely thin and it was decided to perform a ramas grafting procedure prior to implant placement. Under local anesthesia, a full thickness flap was raised, the recipient site and the ramus area were exposed, a bone block of 10 × 15 mm was harvested by using piezotome (Variosurg, NSK, Japan). Decortication of the recipient site was made by using round burr and the bone block was adapted and secured via three titanium screws. In order to avoid soft tissue ingrowth into the existing minimal gap between the bone block and the alveolar bone, the entire surface of the bone block was covered with cross-linked HA gel (Flex Barrier Hyaluronic Acid Gel, Hyadent Bioscience Gmbh, Ransbach-Baumbach, Germany) (**Figure 18**).

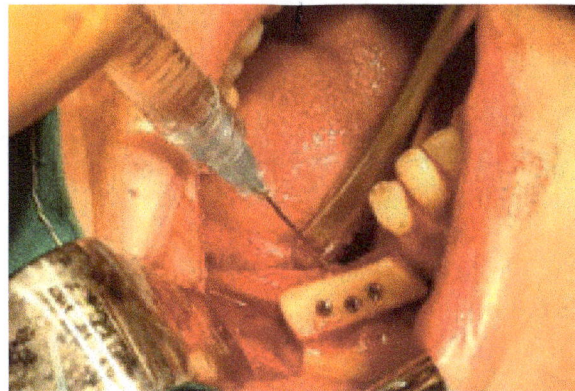

Figure 18. In order to avoid soft tissue ingrowth into the existing minimal gap between the bone block and the alveolar bone, the entire surface of the bone block was covered with cross-linked HA gel.

The postoperative period was uneventful. Three months postoperatively, radiological examination showed successful healing at the grafted site (**Figure 19**) and two implants were inserted into the grafted site (**Figure 20**).

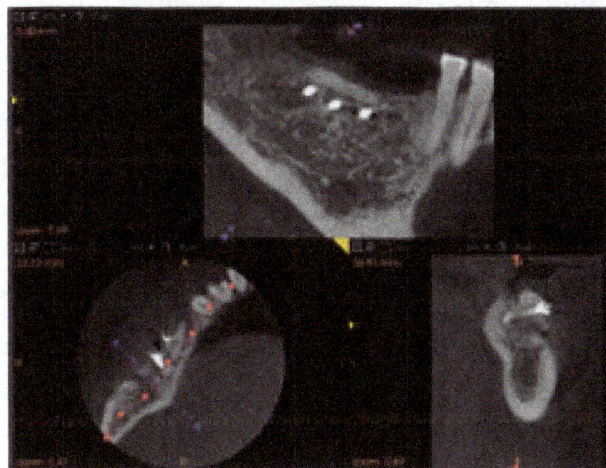

Figure 19. Three months postoperatively, radiological examination showed successful healing at the grafted site.

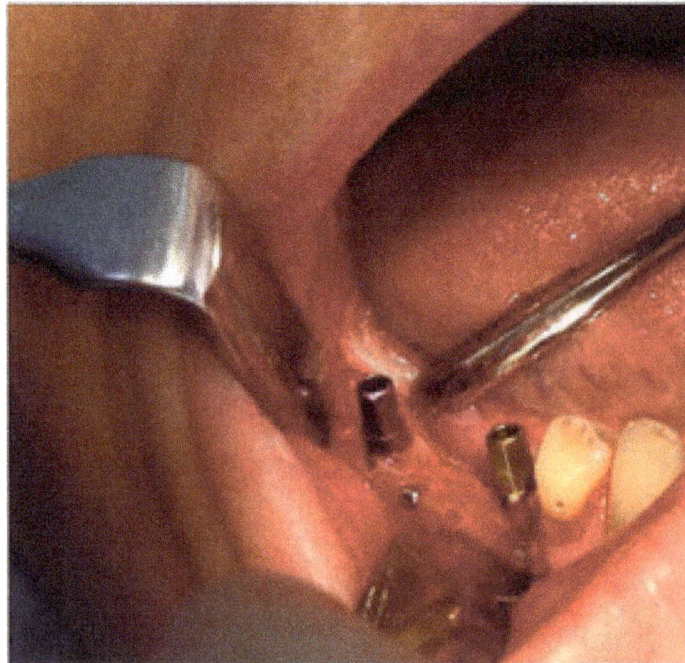

Figure 20. Two implants were placed into the grafted site.

5.5. Ridge splitting

A 44-year-old female patient was admitted due to the difficulties in eating. Clinically and radiographically, her left posterior mandible area was extremely thin and it was decided to perform a ridge splitting procedure prior to implant placement (**Figure 21**).

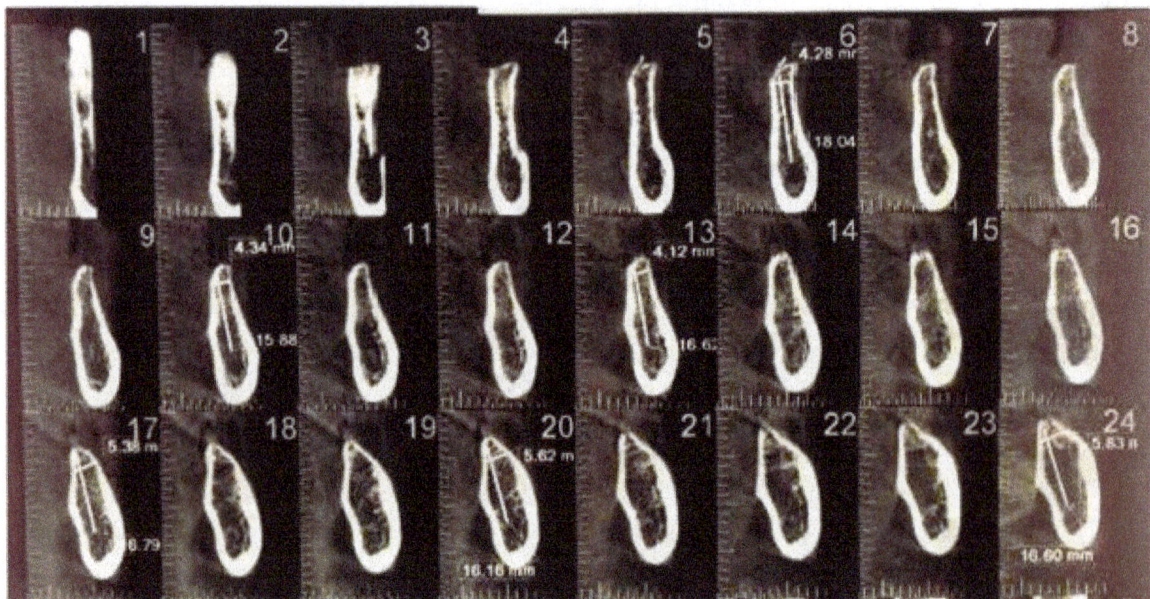

Figure 21. Radiographically, the corresponding area was extremely thin.

Under local anesthesia, a full thickness flap was raised, the recipient site and the ramus area were exposed, the alveolar ridge was decorticated and then splitted via osteotomes (**Figure 22**).

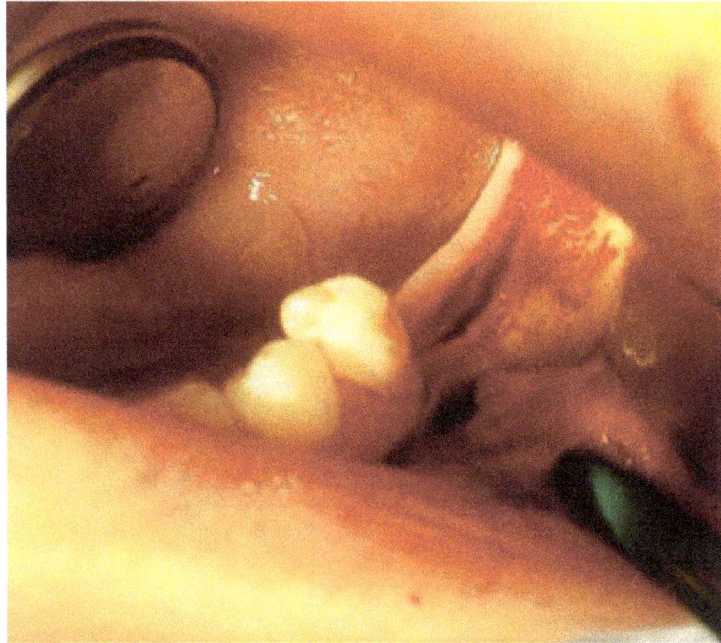

Figure 22. The alveolar ridge was split via osteotomes.

A bone spreader was used to prepare the implant sockets (**Figure 23**).

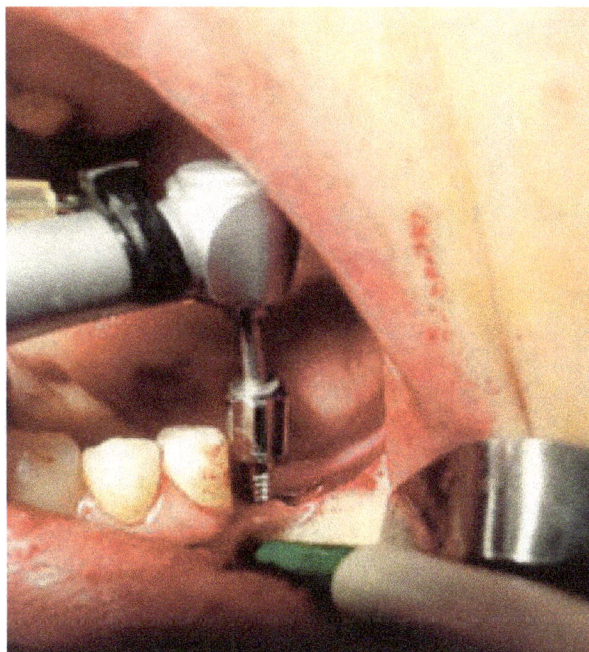

Figure 23. Bone spreader was used to prepare the implant sockets.

Two implants (Bone Trust, Medical Instinct Zahn Implantate, Bovenden, Germany) were inserted into the grafted area (**Figure 24**).

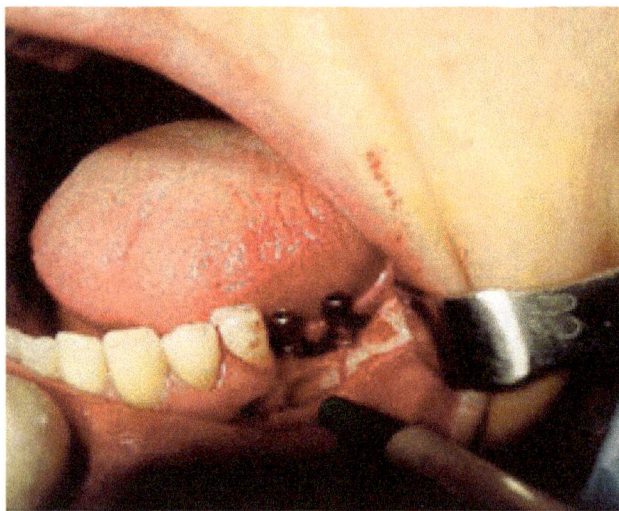

Figure 24. Two implants (Bone Trust, Medical Instinct Zahn Implantate, Bovenden, Germany) were inserted into the grafted area.

The gap between the splitted fragments were grafted with bioactive glass bone graft material (Leonardo, Naturelize, Hirschberg, Germany), which we had mixed with non-cross-linked HA (Tissue Support Hyaluronic Acid Liqui Gel, Hyadent Bioscience Gmbh, Ransbach-Baumbach, Germany) (**Figure 25**).

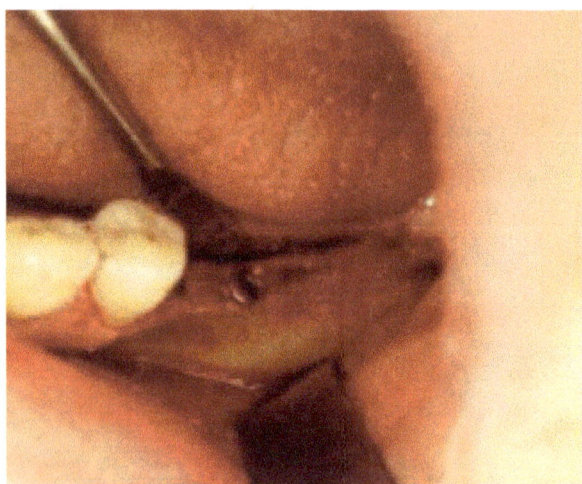

Figure 25. The gap between the splitted fragments were grafted with bioactive glass bone graft material (Leonardo, Naturelize, Hirschberg, Germany), which we had mixed with non-cross-linked hyaluronic acid (Tissue Support Hyaluronic Acid Liqui Gel, Hyadent Bioscience Gmbh, Ransbach-Baumbach, Germany).

In order to avoid soft tissue ingrowth into the existing minimal gap between the bone block and the alveolar bone, the entire surface of the splitted area was covered with cross-linked HA gel (Flex Barrier Hyaluronic Acid Gel, Hyadent Bioscience Gmbh, Ransbach-Baumbach, Germany) (**Figure 26**). The postoperative period was uneventful.

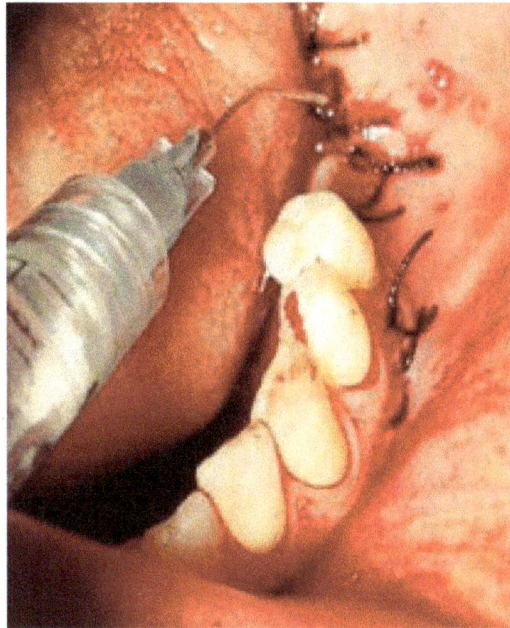

Figure 26. In order to avoid soft tissue ingrowth into the existing minimal gap between the bone block and the alveolar bone, the entire surface of the splitted area was covered with cross-linked HA gel (Flex Barrier Hyaluronic Acid Gel, Hyadent Bioscience Gmbh, Ransbach-Baumbach, Germany) before and after primary closure.

5.6. Filling of the bone defects following removal of oral lesions

A 64-year-old male patient was admitted due to swelling of his upper edentulous right maxilla. Radiographically, a radio-opacity resembling a residual root tip surrounded by a radiolucency was observed (**Figure 27**).

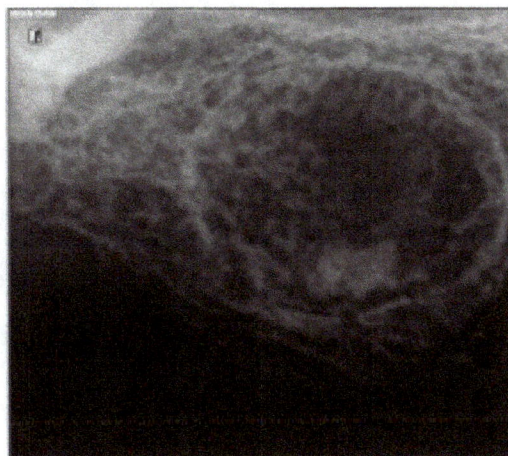

Figure 27. A radio-opacity resembling a residual root tip surrounded by a radiolucency.

Under local anesthesia, a full thickness flap was raised, the corresponding area was exposed (**Figure 28**) and the cyst was curetted.

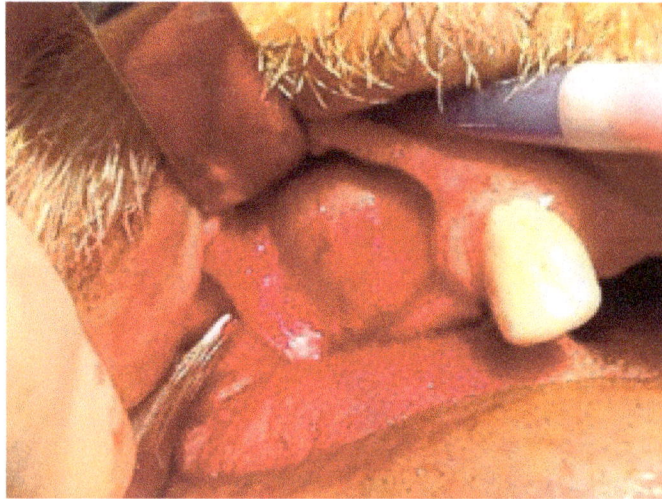

Figure 28. Surgical exposure of the cyst.

The cavity was filled with a bioactive glass bone graft material (Leonardo, Naturelize, Hirschberg, Germany), which we had mixed with non-cross-linked HA (Tissue Support Hyaluronic Acid Liqui Gel, Hyadent Bioscience Gmbh, Ransbach-Baumbach, Germany) extra-orally and the lateral coverage of the augmentation site was made by using cross-linked HA gel (Flex Barrier Hyaluronic Acid Gel, Hyadent Bioscience Gmbh, Ransbach-Baumbach, Germany). On the radiographic examination 2 months postoperatively, particulated structure of the graft material and radio-opaque structure resembling the newly formed bone were observed (**Figure 29**).

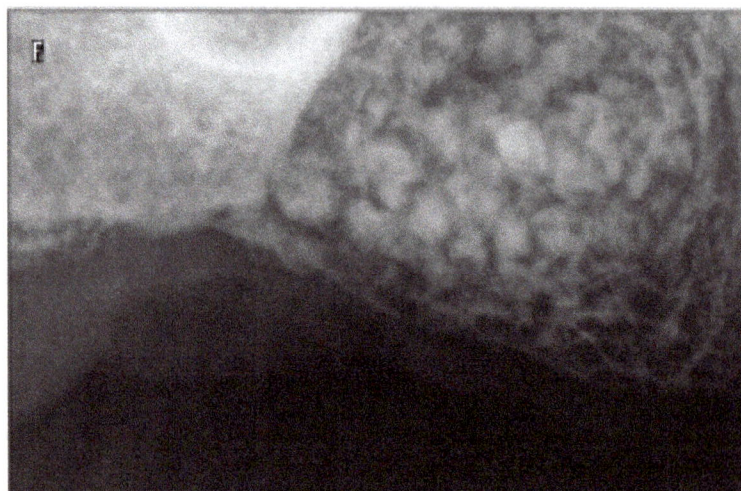

Figure 29. Two months postoperatively, radiological examination showed successful healing and particulated structure of the bone graft material.

The patient underwent implant surgery 3 months after cyst removal (**Figure 30**).

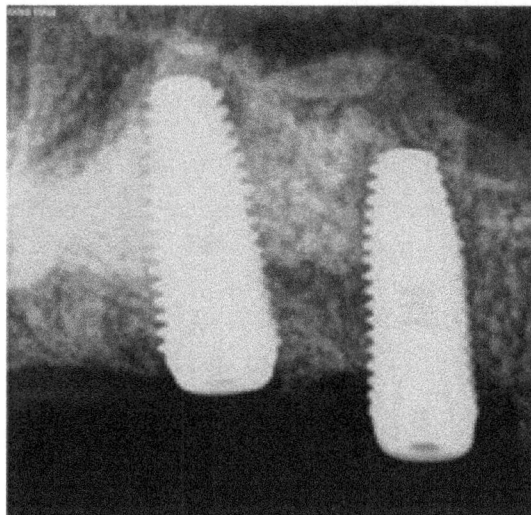

Figure 30. The patient underwent an implant surgery 3 months after cyst removal.

Two implants (Oxy Biomec SRL, Colico, Italy) were placed into the grafted site. As can be seen from our clinical outcomes, HA is a highly promising material for improving therapeutic outcomes for oral implantology.

Author details

Fatih Özan[1*], Metin Şençimen[2], Aydın Gülses[2] and Mustafa Ayna[3]

*Address all correspondence to: dtfatihozan@gmail.com

1 Faculty of Dentistry, Department of Oral and Maxillofacial Surgery, AbantİzzetBaysal University, Bolu, Turkey

2 Department of Dental Sciences, Department of Oral and Maxillofacial Surgery, Gülhane Military Medical Academy, Ankara, Turkey

3 Center for Implant Dentistry, Duisburg, Germany

References

[1] Schropp L, Wenzel A, Kostopoulos L, Karring T: Bone healing and soft tissue contour changes following single-tooth extraction: a clinical and radiographic 12-month prospective study. Int J Periodontics Restorative Dent. 2003; 23: 313-323.

[2] Dahlin C, Gottlow J, Lindhe A, Nyman S: Healing of maxillary and mandibular bone defects using a membrane technique. An experimental study in monkeys. Scand J Plast Reconstr Surg Hand Surg. 1990; 24: 13-19.

[3] Dahlin C, Linde A, Gottlow J, Nyman S: Healing of bone defects by guided tissue regeneration. Plast Reconstr Surg. 1988 ; 81: 672-676.

[4] Dahlin C, Sennerby L, Lekholm U, Linde A, Nyman S: Generation of new bone around titanium implants using a membrane technique: an experimental study in rabbits. Int J Oral Maxillofac Implants. 1989; 4: 19-25.

[5] Urist MR, McLean FC: Recent advances in physiology of bone: Part I. J Bone Joint Surg Am. 1963; 45: 1305-1313.

[6] Murphy KG: Postoperative healing complications associated with Gore-Tex periodontal material. Part I. Incidence and characterization. Int J Periodontics Restorative Dent. 1995; 15: 363-375.

[7] Wang HL, Carroll MJ: Guided bone regeneration using bone grafts and collagen membranes. Quintessence Int. 2001; 32: 504-515.

[8] Baisse E, Piotrowski B, Piantoni P, Brunel G: Action of hyaluronic acid on the wound healing process following extraction. Dent Inf. 2004; 7: 1-9.

[9] Huang L, Cheng YY, Koo PL, Lee KM, Qin L, Cheng JC, Kumpta SM: The effect of hyaluronan on osteoblast proliferation and differentiation in rat calvarial-derived cell cultures. J Biomed Mater Res. 2003; 15; 66A: 880-884.

[10] Peattle RA, Nayate AP, Firpo MA, Shelby J, Fisher RJ, Prestwich GD: Stimulation of in vivo angiogenesis by cytokine-loaded hyaluronic acid hydrogel implants. Biomaterials. 2004; 25(14): 2789-2798.

[11] Chen J, Abatangelo G: Functions of hyaluronan in wound repair. Wound Repair Regen. 1999; 7: 79-89.

[12] Toole BP: Hyaluronan and its binding proteins, the hyaladherins. Curr Opin Cell Biol. 1990; 2: 839-844.

[13] Petersen S, Kaule S, Teske M, Minrath I, Schmitz KP, Sternberg K: Development and in vitro characterization of hyaluronic acid-based coatings for implant-associated local drug delivery systems. J Chem. 2013; 2013(2013):11. Article ID 587875. doi: 10.1155/2013/587875.

[14] Nolon A, Baillie C, Badminton J, Rudralinglam M, Seymour RA: The efficacy of topical hyaluronic acid in the management of recurrent aphthous ulceration. J Oral Pathol Med. 2006; 35: 461-465.

[15] Jentsch H, Pomowski R, Kundt G, Göcke R: Treatment of gingivitis with hyaluronan. J Clin Periodontal. 2003; 30: 159-164.

[16] Mendes RM, Silva GA, Lima MF, Calliari MV, Almeida AP, Alves JB, Ferreira AJ: Sodium hyaluronate accelerates the healing process in tooth sockets of rats. Arch Oral Biol. 2008; 53: 1155-1162.

[17] Mansouri SS, Ghasemi M, Salmani Z, Shams N: Clinical application of hyaluronic acid gel for reconstruction of interdental papilla at the esthetic zone. JIDA. 2013; 25: 152-157.

[18] Claar M: Hyaluronic acid in oral implantology. EDI Case Studies. 2013; 4: 64-68.

[19] Wang HL, Carroll MJ: Guided bone regeneration using bone grafts and collagen membranes. Quintessence Int. 2001; 32: 504-515.

[20] Hitti RA, Kerns DG: Guided bone regeneration in the oral cavity: a review. Open Pathol J. 2011; 5: 33-45.

[21] Marinucci L, Lilli C, Baroni T: In vitro comparison of bioabsorbable and non-resorbable membranes in bone regeneration. J Periodontol. 2001; 72: 753-759.

[22] Blumenthal NM: The use of collagen membranes to guide regeneration of new connective tissue attachment in dogs. J Periodontol. 1988; 59: 830-836.

2

Treatment Protocol for Skeletal Class III Malocclusion in Growing Patients

Jamilian Abdolreza, Khosravi Saeed and
Darnahal Alireza

Abstract

Maxillary deficiency in growing patients with skeletal Class III malocclusion can be treated by either extraoral or intraoral appliances. Extraoral appliances include face mask, reverse chin cup, reverse headgear, and protraction headgear. Intraoral appliances include tongue appliance, fixed tongue appliance, tongue plate, Frankel III, miniplate in combination with Class III elastics, and miniscrew in combination with Class III elastics. Herein, we demonstrate our experience and treatment results in these patients.

Keywords: skeletal Class III malocclusion, maxillary deficiency, orthodontic treatment, growing patients, maxillary retrusion

1. Introduction

Skeletal Class III malocclusion is characterized by mandibular prognathism, maxillary deficiency, or some combination of these two features. The prevalence of Class III malocclusion varies among different ethnic groups. The prevalence in Caucasians ranges between 1% and 4%. A high prevalence has been reported in Asians. Various studies have reported that 4–12% of Chinese and 9–19% of Koreans suffer from Class III malocclusion which is relatively higher than 0.6–1.2% reported for African Americans and 6% reported for the Swedish population [1].

Approximately half of all skeletal Class III malocclusions are reported to result from maxillary deficiency. More precisely, the incidence of Class III malocclusions suffering from maxillary deficiency was reported to be 65–67% [2]. If the mandible of the patients is markedly affected, then the most common treatment would be orthodontics in combination with orthognathic surgery. In this chapter, the main focus of attention will be on maxillary deficiency in growing patients (pseudo-Class III).

In view of the high frequency of maxillary deficiency, maxillary advancement by orthopedic force is considered to be a viable treatment option in growing patients [3, 4]. A number of techniques have been described, including the use of a face mask [5–7], reverse chin cup [8], and direct force application through implants placed in the zygomatic processes [9]. It was also suggested that intentionally ankylosed teeth may be used as abutments for extraoral traction in patients with a severe disturbance in maxillary growth [10]. Miniscrew implants and miniplates have also been used to provide the necessary orthodontic anchorage in these cases [11–14]. The tongue plate and tongue appliance have also been used for the correction of maxillary deficiency in growing patients [15–17]. The mechanism of action associated with these appliances relies upon forward pressure from the tongue, which is transmitted via the appliance to the maxillary dentition and maxilla.

2. Treatment of maxillary deficiency in growing patients

Growing patients with skeletal Class III malocclusion characterized by maxillary deficiency can be treated by either extraoral or intraoral appliances. Extraoral appliances include face mask, reverse chin cup, reverse headgear, and protraction headgear and intraoral appliances include tongue appliance, fixed tongue appliance, tongue plate, Frankel III, miniplate in combination with Class III elastics, and miniscrew in combination with Class III elastics.

2.1. Extraoral appliances

2.1.1. Face mask

Face mask therapy has become a common technique used to correct the developing Class III malocclusion. A literature search will reveal extensive research on face masks and their effects on the nasomaxillary complex. In addition, the experimental studies constantly demonstrate pronounced forward movement of the maxilla due to heavy and continuous protraction forces of face masks [18]. Face masks were first described more than a century ago [19]. Delaire et al.'s [19] face mask promotes midface orthopedic expansion with slight inferior and anterior movement of the maxilla. The protraction face mask provides a direct constant anterior force to the maxilla with downward and backward rotation of the mandible [20]. Nanda introduced a modified protraction headgear that aimed to control the point and direction of force application [21] (**Figure 1**). Similar appliances to the face mask have been proposed by various clinicians and vary slightly from each other but their mechanisms are almost the same. Some of these appliances are reverse headgear, front pull headgear, and protraction headgear among others.

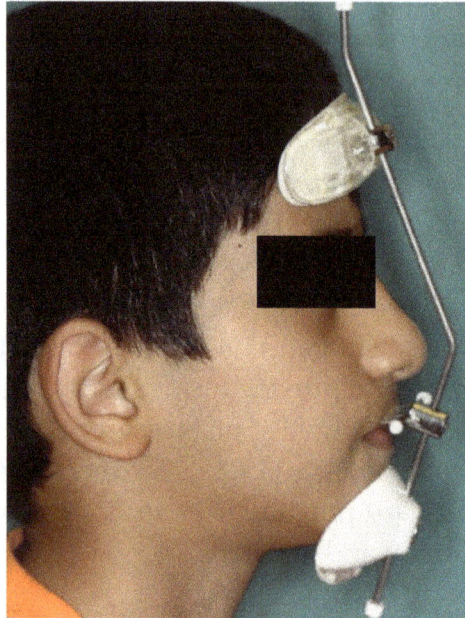

Figure 1. Face mask in situ; note forehead and chin pads, main bar, crossbar, and elastics connecting the crossbar to the maxilla.

2.1.1.1. Limitations

However, one of the problems with face masks is their bulky size and shape, which make it a discouraging choice for children. Patients who wear glasses will be especially more susceptible to discomfort. This discomfort along with the embarrassment caused by the large size, especially for children at school in front of other, may reduce patient compliance. The forehead and the chin are used as areas that support the face mask. Nanda reported that in face mask therapy although the maxilla will translate forward, downward and backward rotations of mandible are unavoidable [21]. The backward and downward rotations of the mandible are unfavorable in patients with vertical growth pattern. On the contrary, this effect may be favorable in patients with a horizontal growth pattern. Face mask would also cause forward movement of the maxillary dentition and lingual movement of the mandibular incisors [8].

2.1.2. Reverse chin cup

The chin cup is an extraoral appliance first introduced by Showkatbakhsh et al. [8, 22]. The reverse chin cup is composed of an upper removable appliance and a custom made porous acrylic chin cup with two vertical arms. The upper removable appliance consists of two Adams clasps on the permanent first molars, two C clasps on the primary canines, and two C clasps on the permanent central incisors. If necessary, the number of C clasps and Adams clasps can be increased for anchorage reinforcement. The end of each arm of the chin cup is bent to form a hook. Two orthodontic latex elastics (recommended: 5/16, heavy elastics) connect the hooks of the palatal canine area of the upper removable appliance to the hooks of reverse chin cup in order to deliver approximately 500 g of force on each side. A high pull head cup is used to hold the reverse chin cup. The patients are instructed to wear the appliance full time except for eating, contact sports, and toothbrushing (**Figure 2**).

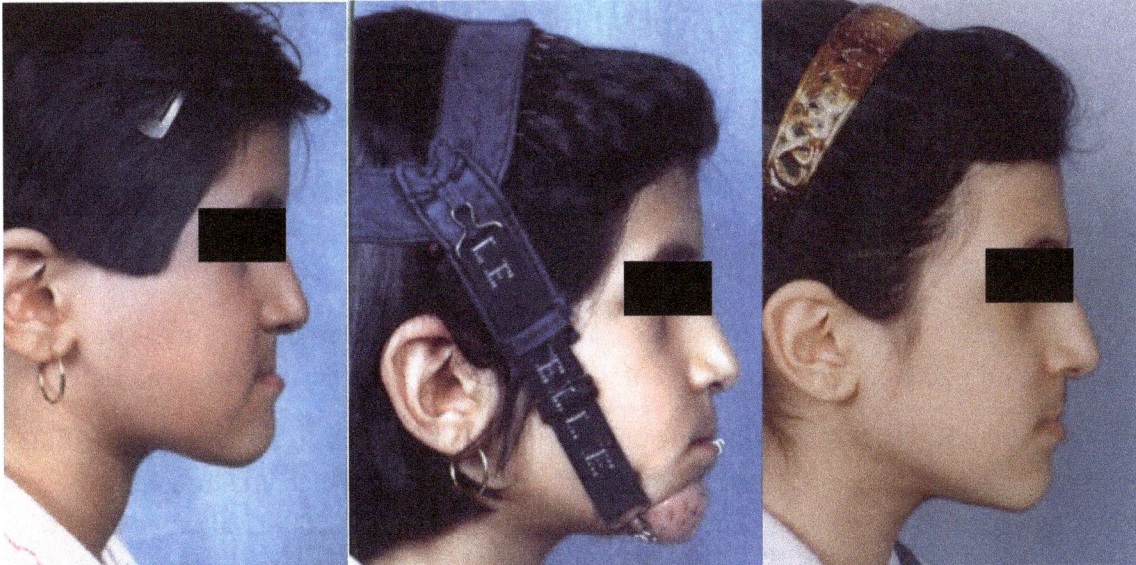

Figure 2. A 6-year-old patient in the mixed dentition with Class III malocclusion and maxillary deficiency. Concave profile was obvious. She had a reverse overjet and underbite. She was treated via reverse chin cup. After 18 months of treatment, her profile improved and a positive overjet was achieved.

The reverse chin cup is very similar to the face mask and is able to produce forward movement of the maxilla in growing patients; however, chin cup may be more favorable for patients due to its smaller size.

2.1.2.1. Limitations

Similar to face masks reverse chin cup is also associated with lingual tipping of the lower incisors and labial tipping of the uppers. Another drawback of the reverse chic cup is backward and downward rotation of the mandible.

2.2. Intraoral appliances

2.2.1. Removable tongue appliance

The tongue appliance is a habit breaker which is constructed via Adams clasps in the first upper molars and C clasps in the anterior teeth in order to increase retention. Three to five separate tongue cribs are placed in the palatal area from canine to canine. These cribs are long enough to cage the tongue and are adjusted to prevent traumatizing the floor of the mouth. A screw is mounted in the midpalatal area to correct bilateral posterior cross bite. The patients are instructed to tighten the screw once per week [15] (**Figure 3**).

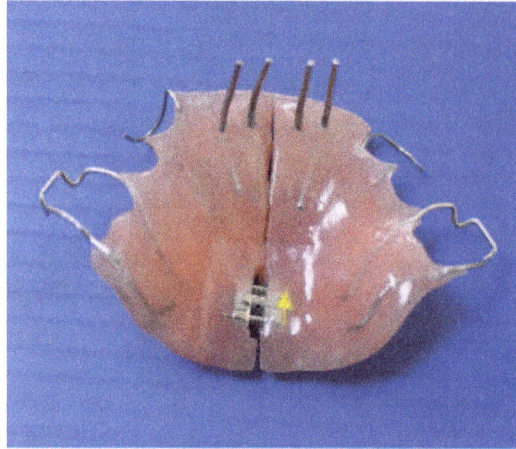

Figure 3. Tongue appliance.

When the tongue appliance is in the mouth, a considerable amount of pressure is transmitted to the deficient maxilla. The mechanism of this force is provided in two ways, namely:

The intermittent force is transferred through the tongue appliance to the deficient nasomaxillary complex via the pressure of the tongue during swallowing which is estimated to be about 5 pounds in each swallow. The frequency of swallowing is about 500–1200 times in 24 h.

Pressure to the tongue appliance transmits considerable force while it is in the rest position. This continuous force of the tongue pushes the maxilla into a forward position.

Physiological position and functional activity of tongue generate these forces. These forces are transmitted by the tongue through the palatal cribs and finally to the nasomaxillary complex. The more anterior the tongue is, the greater the force will be; the more posterior the crib is, the greater the force will be (**Figure 4**).

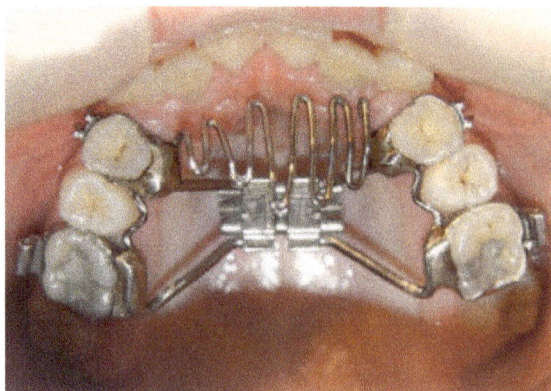

Figure 4. Fixed tongue appliance in situ.

Unlike extraoral appliances such as the face mask and reverse chin cup, the removable tongue appliance has no adverse effects on the mandible and would not cause its backward and downward rotation. Another advantage of this appliance over the other extraoral appliances is that it is less conspicuous and needs less patient compliance.

2.2.1.1. Limitations

The removable tongue appliance will lingualize the lower incisors due to elimination of tongue pressure. In other words, after discontinuing the appliance, the IMPA will be increased and the overjet will be decreased [23]. Another disadvantage of removable tongue appliance is the need for patient cooperation and lack of compliance of which would have negative effects on the final result.

2.2.2. Fixed tongue appliance

In order to remove the need for patient compliance in removable tongue appliances, Showkatbakhsh et al. designed a new appliance called the "fixed tongue appliance" [24]. Fixed tongue appliances consist of a Hyrax® mounted on the first maxillary molars and premolars; a few curved cribs are soldered to the anterior side of the Hyrax® (**Figure 4**). The patient is instructed to activate the screw of the Hyrax® by making 1/4 of a turn at the beginning of each week. Fixed tongue appliance is a habit breaker used in conjunction with the Hyrax® for a different purpose other than its common application. The Hyrax® screw is for the purpose of loosening the maxillary sutures and extending the width of the maxillary arch and thus creating a better intermaxillary relationship. This expansion facilitates anterior displacement of the maxilla. When the fixed tongue appliance is in the mouth, a considerable amount of pressure is transmitted to the deficient maxilla through the cribs of the appliance. The mechanism of this force is similar to the removable tongue appliance (**Figures 5** and **6**). The fixed tongue appliance is used for the correction of skeletal problems and further treatment by fixed orthodontics is required for dental problems (**Figure 7**).

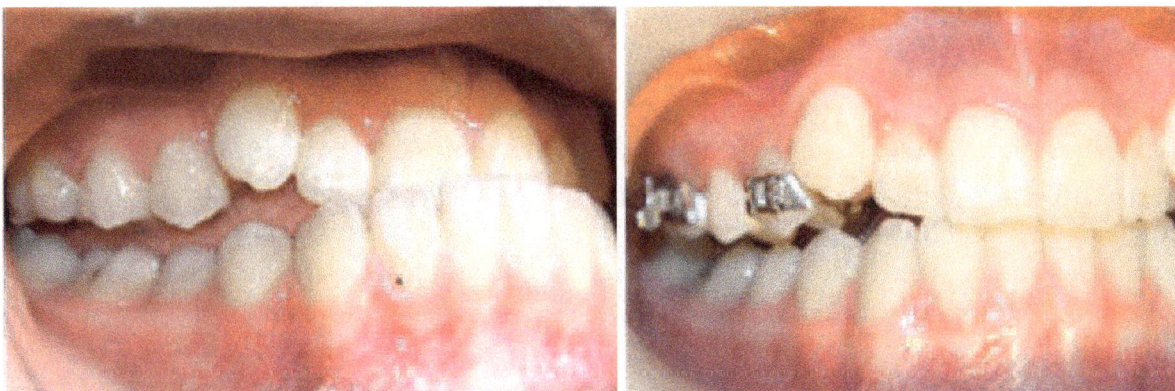

Figure 5. A 12-year-old girl with maxillary deficiency in the late mixed dentition and Class III molar and canine relationships. Skeletal problems of the patient were corrected by means of a fixed tongue appliance

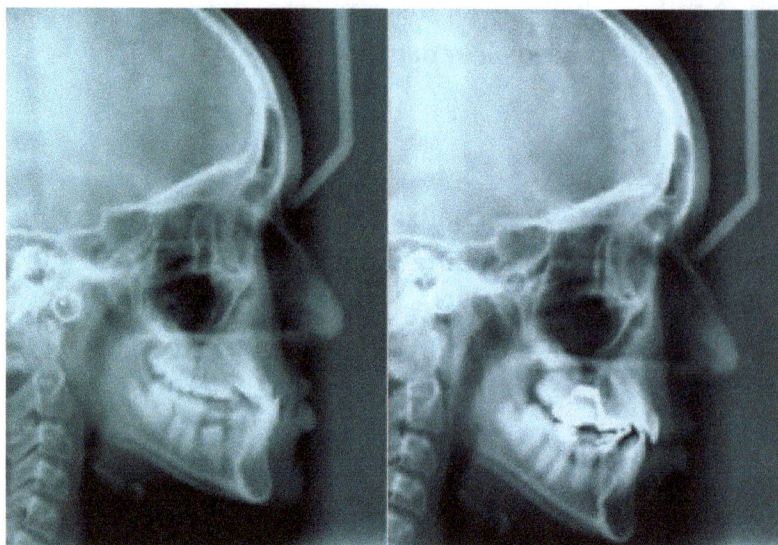

Figure 6. Pre- and post-treatment lateral cephalograms of the same patient.

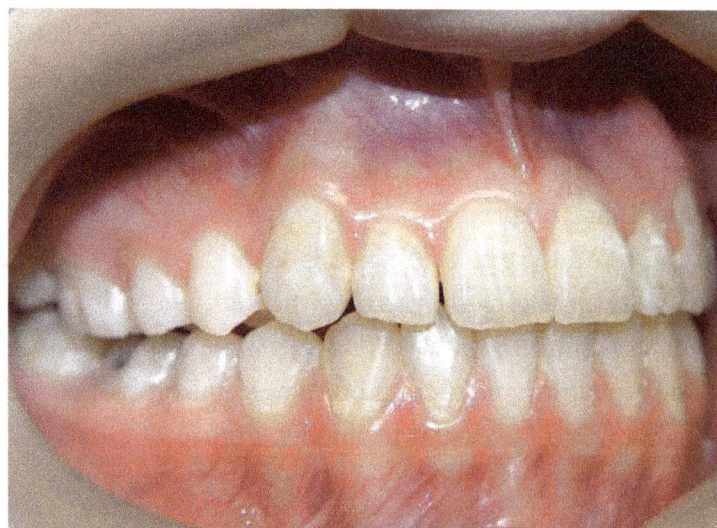

Figure 7. The occlusion of the same patient treated by fixed orthodontics.

One of the advantages of the fixed tongue appliance is that patient's cooperation is not needed. The vertical length of the cribs should be designed and adjusted in a way to avoid traumatizing the floor of the mouth. The main advantage of the fixed tongue appliance over the face mask is that the fixed tongue appliance does not cause backward rotation of the mandible; thus, it can be used in long-face patients, while the cup of the face mask results in backward rotation of the mandible and can have unfavorable effects in long-face patients [25].

2.2.2.1. Limitations

The fixed tongue appliance has one disadvantage. It will lingualize the lower incisors due to elimination of pressure of the tongue on them. However, removal of the fixed tongue appliance will restore the pressure of the tongue on the lower incisors and will consequently result in the increase of the IMPA.

2.2.3. Tongue plate

The tongue plate is a tightly fitting and well-retained upper removable appliance fabricated with Adams clasps on the upper first permanent molars and C clasps placed on the upper primary canines [17]. Additional C clasps can be added if more retention is needed. An acrylic plate was mounted posterior to the upper incisors. The patients were instructed to wear the appliance full time except for eating, contact sports, and toothbrushing (**Figure 8**).

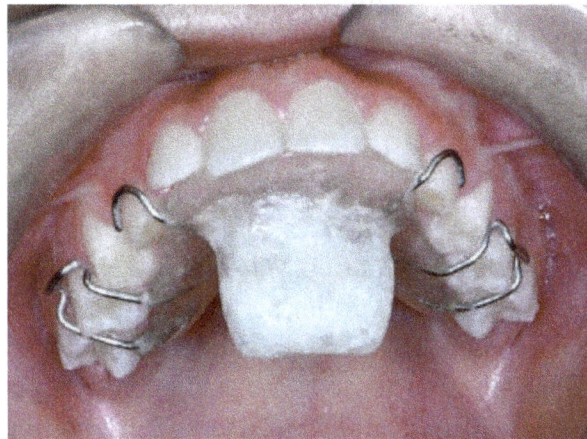

Figure 8. Tongue plate in situ.

The mechanism of action of the tongue plate is very similar to the fixed and removable tongue appliance. The force of the tongue during swallowing and resting is transferred through the tongue plate to the deficient nasomaxillary complex. The force of the tongue which is considerable is caged behind the acrylic plate and moves the maxilla in a forward position. The rounded surface of the plate and its softened edges make it undamaging for the tongue. In addition, it is designed and adjusted in a way to avoid traumatizing the floor of the mouth.

The disadvantages of the tongue plate are similar to those of fixed and removable tongue appliances in that it also lingualizes the lower incisors.

2.2.4. Frankel III appliance

The Frankel III appliance is a removable appliance used to stimulate the growth of the upper jaw and move it forward. The appliance was first designed by Professor Frankel and is composed of wire and four acrylic parts: two vestibular shields and two upper labial pads [26]. The vestibular shields extend from the depth of the mandibular vestibule to the height of the maxillary vestibule. These shields act to remove the restrictive forces created by the buccinator and associated facial muscles against the lateral surfaces of the alveoli and the buccal dentition. The appliance allows the maxillary molars to erupt and move mesially while holding the lower molars in place vertically and anteroposteriorly; it also tips the maxillary anterior teeth facially and retracts the anterior mandibular teeth. Vertical movement of the maxillary molar will help rotate the chin down and back to improve facial appearance.

2.2.4.1. Limitations

The Frankel III appliance requires a lengthy treatment time and excellent patient cooperation.

2.3. Skeletal anchorage

Recently dental implants, miniplates, and modified fixation screws have become popular for bone anchorage in orthodontics. These temporary skeletal anchorage devices (TAD) are smaller than extraoral appliances and require short healing periods [27]. Various techniques have been developed to use miniplates and miniscrews as temporary anchorage devices. De Clerck et al. treated a series of Class III cases with orthopedic traction on miniplates [12].

2.3.1. Miniplate in combination with Class III elastics

Showkatbakhsh et al. [13] used Class III elastics connected from two mandibular miniplates to an upper removable appliance to treat an 11-year-old boy with maxillary deficiency. Plates for orthodontic anchorage were placed under local anesthesia in the canine areas of the mandible by a maxillofacial surgeon. The ideal position for miniplate insertion was evaluated by using a panoramic radiograph in order to avoid damage to the roots of the adjacent teeth and mental foramen. A tightly fitting and well-retained upper removable appliance was fabricated with two Adams clasps on the upper first permanent molars. Each of the Adams clasps had a loop which was used for retaining the elastics. A labial bow was also used on the anterior teeth for retention. A maxillary posterior bite plate was used to disocclude the upper and lower jaws. Orthodontic latex elastics (3/16″ heavy size) were connected from the hooks of the miniplates to the Adams clasps of the removable appliance to generate approximately 500 g of anterior retraction. The patient was instructed to wear the appliance full time except for eating, contact sports, and toothbrushing; he was also told to change the elastics every day (**Figure 9**). After 10 months of active treatment, a positive overjet and Class I buccal segments were achieved and the anterior cross bite of the patient was corrected (**Figures 10** and **11**).

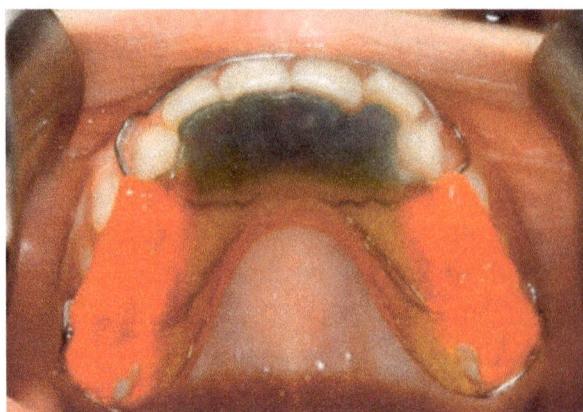

Figure 9. Miniplate in situ.

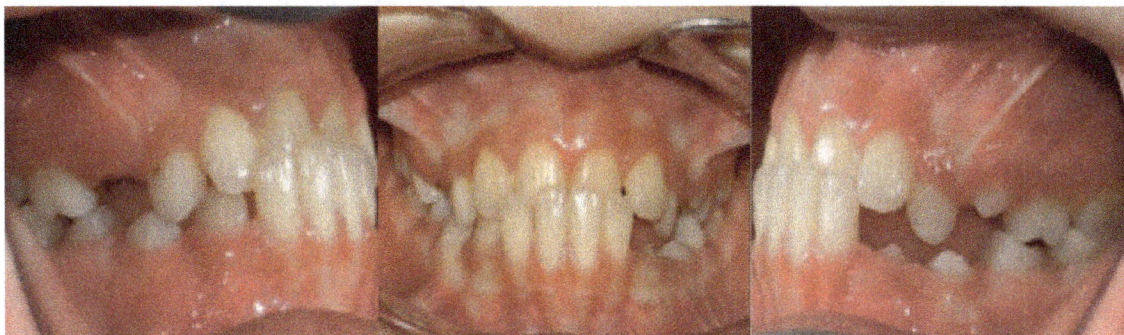

Figure 10. Pretreatment photos of an 11-year-old boy with pseudoprognathism (maxillary deficiency).

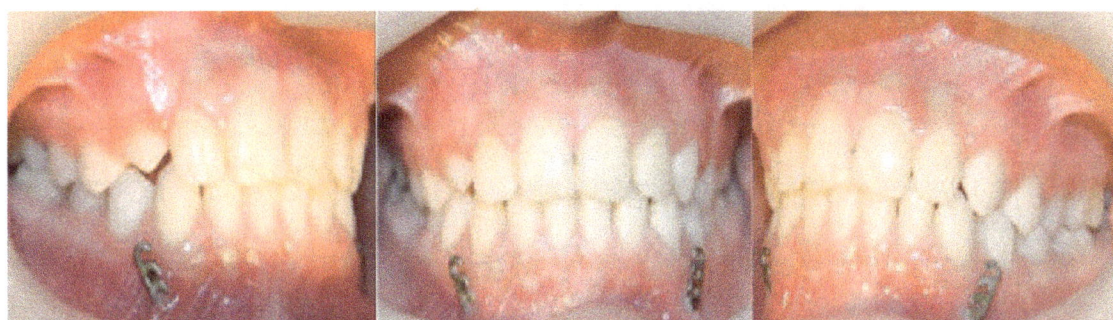

Figure 11. Posttreatment photos of the same patient treated by miniplates and Class III elastics.

2.3.1.1. Limitations

The need for minor surgery for inserting and removing the miniplates is their biggest disadvantage. Moreover, since the surgery involves flap elevation, it must be done by a maxillofacial surgeon under local anesthesia. Difficult oral hygiene around the appliance is another disadvantage of miniplates.

2.3.2. Miniscrews in combination with Class III elastics

Ease of placement, often by orthodontists themselves, has made miniscrews very popular. When used as orthodontic anchorage, they also have the advantage of fewer adverse effects and lower operational costs than tooth implants. Recently, Jamilian et al. used titanium alloy miniscrews along with Class III elastics for forward positioning of the maxilla of a patient with maxillary deficiency. In order to do so, self-drilling titanium alloy Jeil™ miniscrews (Jeil Medical Corp., Seoul, Korea; 1.6 mm diameter, 8 mm length) were placed under local anesthesia into the buccal alveolar bone between the mandibular canine and first premolar roots on both sides. The ideal position for screw insertion was evaluated by using a panoramic radiograph in order to avoid damage to the roots of the adjacent teeth and mental foramen. A tightly fitting and well-retained upper removable appliance was fabricated with Adams clasps on the upper first permanent molars and premolars. C clasps were placed on the upper permanent canines and central incisors. Orthodontic latex elastics (5/16″ medium size) were connected from the miniscrews to the Adams clasps of the removable appliance to generate about 450 g of anterior retraction. The patient was instructed to wear the elastics all the time, except for eating and to change the elastics every day. In order to retain these elastics, the Adams clasps on the molars and premolars were bent to form four loops; however in order to achieve optimal traction, the elastics were only connected to the loops adjacent to the molars (**Figure 12**).

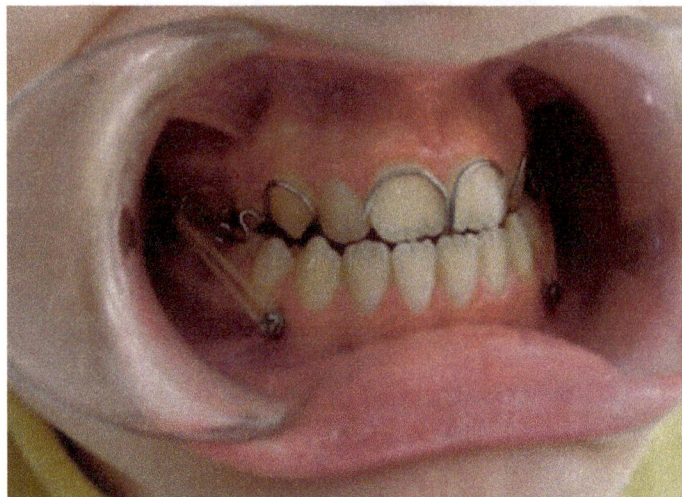

Figure 12. Miniscrews and Class III elastics.

An expansion screw was placed in the midpalatal area of the upper removable appliance and the patient was instructed to turn the screw once a week in order to correct the posterior cross bites. Two Z-springs were inserted in the upper removable appliance to correct the cross bite on the lateral incisors (**Figure 13**).

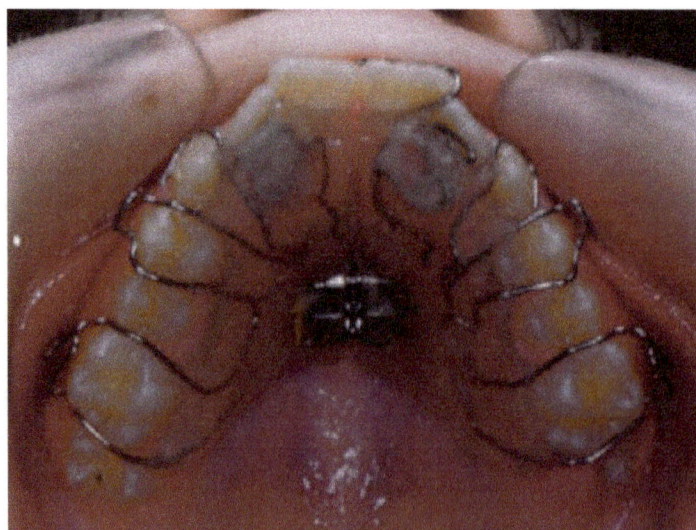

Figure 13. Expansion of the maxillary arch.

After 8 months of active treatment, a positive overjet and Class I buccal segments were achieved and the cross bites were corrected (**Figures 14** and **15**).

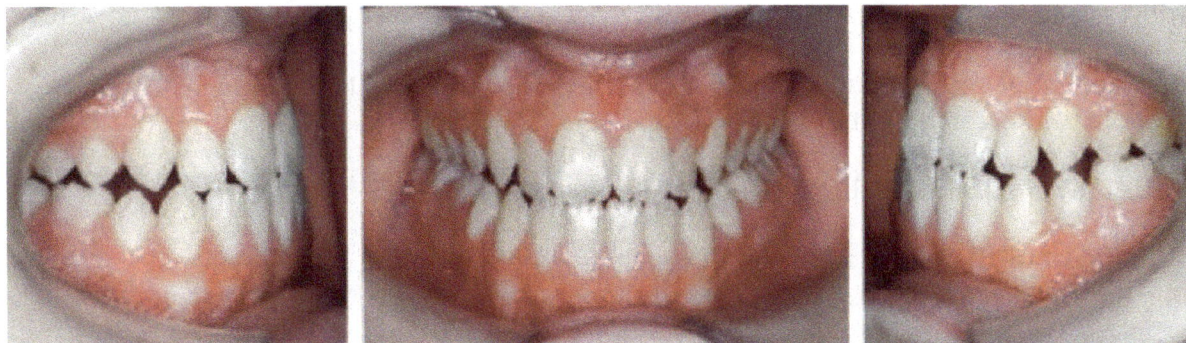

Figure 14. Pretreatment photographs of a 12-year-old boy with maxillary deficiency.

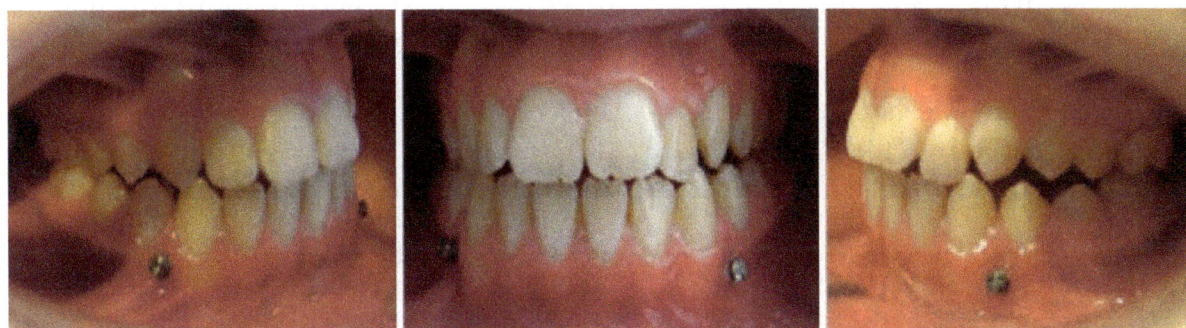

Figure 15. Post-treatment photographs of the same patient.

2.3.2.1. Limitations

The limitations of miniscrews include a high risk of failure when placed in unattached gingiva, screw loosening, tooth root injury when placed in keratinized mucosa, and limited amount and direction of tooth movement depending on the position of the miniscrews.

3. Conclusion

In growing patients with maxillary deficiency, maxillary advancement by orthopedic forces may be considered to be a viable treatment option. A number of techniques have been described, both intraoral and extraoral as well as direct force application through implants placed in the zygomatic processes with good results.

Author details

Jamilian Abdolreza[1*], Khosravi Saeed[2] and Darnahal Alireza[3]

*Address all correspondence to: info@jamilian.net

1 Department of Orthodontics, Islamic Azad University, Tehran Dental Branch, Cranio Maxillofacial Research Centre, Tehran, Iran

2 Tehran University of Medical Sciences, Tehran, Iran

3 Tehran Dental Branch, Islamic Azad University, Tehran, Iran

References

[1] Ngan PW, Sung J-H. Chapter treatment strategies for developing and nondeveloping Class III malocclusions. In Nanda R editor. Esthetics and Biomechanics in Orthodontics, Second Edition. St Louis: WB Saunders.

[2] Ellis E, 3rd, McNamara JA, Jr. Components of adult Class III open-bite malocclusion. Am J Orthod 1984;86:277–290.

[3] Arman A, Toygar TU, Abuhijleh E. Profile changes associated with different orthopedic treatment approaches in class III malocclusions. Angle Orthod 2004;74:733–740.

[4] Maspero C, Galbiati G, Perillo L, Favero L, Giannini L. Orthopaedic treatment efficiency in skeletal Class III malocclusions in young patients: RME-face mask versus TSME. Eur J Paediatr Dent 2012;13:225–230.

[5] Delaire J, Verdon P. The use of heavy postero-anterior extraoral forces by an orthopedic mask in the treatment of dentomaxillary sequellae of labiomaxillopalatal clefts. Chir Pediatr 1983;24:315–322.

[6] Jamilian A, Showkatbakhsh R, Taban T. The effects of fixed and removable face masks on maxillary deficiencies in growing patients. Orthodontics (Chic.) 2012;13:e37–43.

[7] Perillo L, Vitale M, Masucci C, D'Apuzzo F, Cozza P, Franchi L. Comparisons of two protocols for the early treatment of Class III dentoskeletal disharmony. Eur J Orthod 2015;38:51–56

[8] Showkatbakhsh R, Jamilian A, Ghassemi M, Ghassemi A, Taban T, Imani Z. The effects of facemask and reverse chin cup on maxillary deficient patients. J Orthod 2012;39:95–101.

[9] Singer SL, Henry PJ, Rosenberg I. Osseointegrated implants as an adjunct to facemask therapy: a case report. Angle Orthod 2000;70:253–262.

[10] Kokich VG, Shapiro PA, Oswald R, Koskinen-Moffett L, Clarren SK. Ankylosed teeth as abutments for maxillary protraction: a case report. Am J Orthod 1985;88:303–307.

[11] Jamilian A, Showkatbakhsh R. Treatment of maxillary deficiency by miniscrew implants—a case report. J Orthod 2010;37:56–61.

[12] De Clerck HJ, Cornelis MA, Cevidanes LH, Heymann GC, Tulloch CJ. Orthopedic traction of the maxilla with miniplates: a new perspective for treatment of midface deficiency. J Oral Maxillofac Surg 2009;67:2123–2129.

[13] Showkatbakhsh R, Jamilian A, Behnaz M. Treatment of maxillary deficiency by miniplates: a case report. ISRN Surg 2011;2011:854924.

[14] Jamilian A, Haraji A, Showkatbakhsh R, Valaee N. The effects of miniscrew with class III traction in growing patients with maxillary deficiency. Int J Orthod Milwaukee 2011;22:25–30.

[15] Jamilian A, Showkatbakhsh R. The effect of tongue appliance on the maxilla in Class III malocclusion due to maxillary deficiency. Int J Orthod Milwaukee 2009;20:11–14.

[16] Showkatbakhsh R, Jamilian A. A novel method of maxillary deficiency treatment by tongue plate—a case report. Int J Orthod Milwaukee 2011;22:31–34.

[17] Showkatbakhsh R, Toumarian L, Jamilian A, Sheibaninia A, Mirkarimi M, Taban T. The effects of face mask and tongue plate on maxillary deficiency in growing patients: a randomized clinical trial. J Orthod 2013;40:130–136.

[18] Cha KS. Skeletal changes of maxillary protraction in patients exhibiting skeletal class III malocclusion: a comparison of three skeletal maturation groups. Angle Orthod 2003;73:26–35.

[19] Delaire J, Verdon P, Lumineau JP, Cherga-Negrea A, Talmant J, Boisson M. Some results of extra-oral tractions with front-chin rest in the orthodontic treatment of class 3 maxillomandibular malformations and of bony sequelae of cleft lip and palate. Rev Stomatol Chir Maxillofac 1972;73:633–642.

[20] Roberts CA, Subtelny JD. An American Board of Orthodontics case report. Use of the face mask in the treatment of maxillary skeletal retrusion. Am J Orthod Dentofacial Orthop 1988;93:388–394.

[21] Nanda R. Biomechanical and clinical considerations of a modified protraction headgear. Am J Orthod 1980;78:125–139.

[22] Showkatbakhsh R, Jamilian A. A novel approach in treatment of maxillary deficiency by reverse chin cup. Int J Orthod Milwaukee 2010;21:27–31.

[23] Showkatbakhsh R, Jamilian A, Taban T, Golrokh M. The effects of face mask and tongue appliance on maxillary deficiency in growing patients: a randomized clinical trial. Prog Orthod 2012;13:266–272.

[24] Showkatbakhsh R, Jamilian A, Ghassemi M, Ghassemi A, Shayan A. Maxillary deficiency treatment by fixed tongue appliance — a case report. Int J Orthod Milwaukee 2013;24:31–34.

[25] Showkatbakhsh R, Jamilian A, Behnaz M, Ghassemi M, Ghassemi A. The short-term effects of face mask and fixed tongue appliance on maxillary deficiency in growing patients — a randomized clinical trial. Int J Orthod Milwaukee 2015;26:33–38.

[26] McNamara JA, Jr., Huge SA. The functional regulator (FR-3) of Frankel. Am J Orthod 1985;88:409–424.

[27] Cevidanes L, Baccetti T, Franchi L, McNamara JA, Jr., De Clerck H. Comparison of two protocols for maxillary protraction: bone anchors versus face mask with rapid maxillary expansion. Angle Orthod 2010;80:799–806.

3

Bone Regeneration in Implant Dentistry: Role of Mesenchymal Stem Cells

Ruggero Rodriguez y Baena, Silvana Rizzo,
Antonio Graziano and Saturnino Marco Lupi

Abstract

This chapter focuses on a review of the activity of non-embryonic mesenchymal stem cells used to regenerate jaw bones in dentistry. Recent research of non-embryonic stem cells provides new possibilities for noninvasively obtaining new autologous bone from stem cells provided by various tissues from the same patient. Disaggregation of biologic tissue harvested from the patients during surgery permits extraction of stem cells from a small sample of connective tissue obtained from the patient's lingual mucosa or from the postextraction surgical site where the endosseous implant will be inserted.

Keywords: Bone regeneration, mesenchymal stem cells, scaffold, micrografts, socket preservation

1. Bone regeneration in implant dentistry

1.1. Bone components

Bone is formed by organic and inorganic components. Two-thirds of the volume comprises inorganic salts, including calcium, phosphate, carbonate, citrate, and hydroxyl ions (magnesium, sodium, and fluoride) in the form of crystals of hydroxyapatite [1]. The organic portion comprises 99% collagen type I and growth factors, such as osteocalcin, osteonectin, phosphoproteins, proteoglycans, and bone morphogenetic proteins [2].

Bone also includes cellular components, such as pre-osteoblasts, osteoblasts, osteocytes, and osteoclasts. Osteoblasts arise from mesenchymal pluripotent cells, which are cuboidal mononuclear cells located along the bony margins, and are able to form new bone tissue. About 10–20% of osteoblasts are trapped within the matrix they produce by developing into osteocytes, which are considered mature osteoblasts. Osteocytes are smaller than osteoblasts, and have a higher nucleus-to-cytoplasm ratio and a larger number of extensions that allow for intercellular communication. Osteocytes are likely the cells responsible for bone regeneration [3]. Osteoclasts are large multinucleated cells that are polarized, have an average lifespan of 15–20 days, and are derived from bone marrow monocytes [4]. Osteoclasts facilitate bone resorption by reducing the surrounding pH.

1.1.1. Stem cells—mesenchymal stem cells

Stem cells are characterized by their ability to renew by cell division and to differentiate into a diverse range of specialized cell types. The two broad types of mammalian stem cells are embryonic stem cells, which are found in blastocysts, and adult stem cells, which are found in adult tissues such as the bone marrow. In adult organisms, stem cells give rise to progenitor cells that act as a repair system for the body by replenishing specialized cells and tissues. Because adult stem cells are obtained from a developed organism, their use in research and therapy is not as controversial as that of embryonic stem cells, which entail the destruction of an embryo [5].

Mesenchymal stem cells (MSCs) are multipotent adult stem cells with unique biologic properties that are typically associated with their mesodermal lineage (adipogenic, chondrogenic, osteogenic, or myogenic) [6–8]. MSCs were first discovered in 1968 by Friedenstein et al. [9], and are defined as adherent fibroblast-like cells that reside in the bone marrow and are capable of differentiating into bone. MSCs and an adequate blood supply are essential for the bone deposition process and healing. MSCs also contribute to the homeostasis of various tissues, including bone, in adults [10].

MSCs can be expanded in vitro for several passages, are easily accessible, and possess minimal immunogenic or tumorigenic risks, and are thus an excellent cell source of stem cells used in dental, craniofacial, and orthopedic regenerative surgery [11].

In 2006, the International Society for Cellular Therapy established the following definition of MSCs [12]:

1.   Cells that are adherent to plastic under standard tissue-culture conditions;

2.   Cells that are positive for surface markers CD105, CD73, and CD90, but negative for CD34, CD45, CD14, or CD11b, CD79a, or CD19, and human leukocyte antigen-D-related (HLA)-DR surface molecules;

3.   Cells with the capacity to differentiate into osteoblasts, chondrocytes, and adipocytes;

MSCs, which represent ~10% of human stem cells, are rare and heterogeneous; they are part of the connective tissue and support hemopoiesis [13]. MSCs can be expanded in vitro and rapidly reach the desired cell counts for use in vivo [14].

Despite having some common features, MSCs have different characteristics depending on the tissue of origin. MSCs can be isolated from several different tissues, including bone marrow [15], placenta, cord blood [16], adipose tissue [17], muscle [18], periosteum [19], synovium [20], deciduous teeth [21], and brain, kidney, heart, epidermis, and periodontal ligaments [22–24]. Among these, bone marrow and adipose tissue are the most commonly used sources of MSCs because of their relative ease of harvesting. MSCs can differentiate into osteoblasts, adipocytes, chondrocytes, myoblasts, cardiomyocytes, hepatocytes, neurons, astrocytes, endothelial cells, fibroblasts, and stromal cells [25].

2. Bone regeneration

Since Horwitz et al. [26] first demonstrated that MSCs can improve osteogenesis in children with osteogenesis imperfecta, the role of MSCs in bone formation and regeneration has been intensively studied. Studies performed in several animal models revealed that the transplantation of MSCs improves bone regeneration and healing of bony defects [27, 28]. The therapeutic options clinically available for bone reconstruction and regeneration, however, are often unsatisfactory due to morbidity at the donor site or the complexity of allograft procedures.

Bone regeneration in maxillofacial reconstruction is one of the most important applications of MSCs [29]. The repair of craniofacial bone defects remains a challenge, however, and the results depend on the size of the defect, the quality of the soft tissues that cover the defect, and the reconstructive techniques used. In Europe, ~1.5 million patients undergo craniofacial reconstructions annually; ~20% of them continue to experience functional deficiency despite the intervention, and 30,000 patients per year develop donor-site morbidity following oral and maxillofacial reconstruction [30].

Traditional bone regeneration techniques involve autologous, homologous, heterologous, or allogeneic grafts. Autologous bone grafts are considered the best option for damaged tissue repair because of the low risk of immunogenicity or disease transmission compared with allografts (genetically different donors from the same species) or xenografts (donors from another species). Autologous bone grafts are limited due to the scarcity of available autologous tissue for repairing larger bone defects, donor-site morbidity, and potential wound-based infections, as well as the prolonged operative times. In addition, autologous bone grafts require additional surgical procedures, which increase the risk of both donor-site morbidity and significant resorption [31]. Alternative therapies continue to be explored [32], and researchers are attempting to identify the best material for bone regeneration.

Bone regeneration following the use of stem cells occurs through two mechanisms: a direct mechanism, which comprises the integration and differentiation into tissue-specific cells, and begins when transplanted cells take root in the target tissue [33]; and an indirect mechanism, which involves paracrine effects [34].

Differentiation of MSCs into osteoblasts was demonstrated in vitro by cultivating the cells in the presence of ascorbic acid, inorganic phosphate (beta-glycerophosphate), and dexamethasone. In vivo studies suggest that transplanted adult stem cells can integrate into tissues that are different from those of the donor and, in some cases, contribute to their regeneration [35]. Demonstrating the in vivo differentiation of implanted cells is challenging, and researchers often assume that differentiation is the result of interactions between grafted cells and host-site cells, but the capacity of MSCs to release a number of trophic factors could also explain their therapeutic benefit.

Some recent reports suggest that the therapeutic properties of paracrine factors are a common feature of stem cells [36]. The paracrine effect could contribute to bone regeneration via the secretion of trophic and angiogenic molecules such as angiopoietin (Ang)-1, Ang-2, Ang-like-1, Ang-like-2, Ang-like-3, Ang-like-4, vascular endothelial growth factor (VEGF), and fibroblast growth factor-2. These molecules can activate local MSCs, promote tissue regeneration and angiogenesis [37], and inhibit fibrosis, apoptosis, and inflammation [38, 39]. They also have neurogenic, neuroprotective, and synaptogenic effects [40, 41]. Because the survival and differentiation of MSCs at the site of the lesion is limited, paracrine signaling is considered to be the primary mechanism of their therapeutic effects [42]. This hypothesis is supported by in vitro and in vivo studies showing that many cell types respond to paracrine signaling from MSCs, which leads to the modulation of a large number of cellular responses, such as survival, proliferation, migration, and gene expression [39].

The secretion of bioactive factors is thought to play a critical role in the paracrine activity of MSCs. These factors and cytokines can be collected in a conditioned medium (CM), which, when transplanted into animal models of different diseases, has effects that are similar to those exerted by MSCs and can increase the tissue-repair process in acute myocardial infarction [43], wound healing [44, 45], and neuroprotection [46]. Encouraging results have also been obtained following the graft of MSCs obtained from the bone marrow cleft at the level of the maxillary sinus and alveolar schisis [47, 48].

Preliminary studies of bone regeneration used MSC populations that were not expanded from bone marrow due to the reduced number of MSCs in the bone marrow (0.01% of the bone marrow cell population). The use of unexpanded MSCs, however, produced unpredictable results [49], and later advances made it possible to cultivate and characterize MSCs. The osteogenic potential of expanded and purified MSCs has been studied extensively, but with mixed results [50, 51]. Factors that may affect the results relate to the donor site, blood supply, and inadequate osteoblastic differentiation of the implanted cells.

In summary, stem cells are effective for tissue regeneration and future research is warranted despite the low number of clinical studies compared to those in preclinical animal models. The use of MSCs is still limited because of their low accessibility, difficult collection, and poor long-term stability. Stem cells are used mainly in combination with scaffolds or biomaterials to improve their efficacy and stability. Scaffold material is often used to provide mechanical support and as a substrate for cell attachment, proliferation, and differentiation. Regardless of the scaffold used for bone reconstruction, however, bone healing depends mainly on two pivotal factors: the capacity to recruit progenitor cells to the injury site and the presence of healthy vasculature near the injury site. Researchers have identified several different tissue types that can be considered valid MSC donors.

2.1. Dental pulp stem cells

Dental pulp is a source of neural crest-derived stem cells that is easily accessible and characterized by low morbidity after collection [52, 53]. Dental pulp comprises both ectodermic and mesenchymal components, and is divided into four layers (outer to inner). The external layer is made up of odontoblast-producing dentin. The second layer, called the "cell-free zone," is poor in cells and rich in extracellular matrix. The third layer, called the "cell-rich zone," contains progenitor cells that exhibit plasticity and pluripotent capabilities [52]. Finally, the inner layer comprises the vascular area and nerve plexus.

In the context of the oral and maxillofacial area, dental pulp stem cells (DPSCs) and periosteal stem cells may be optimal alternatives to MSCs and display high potential for differentiating into a variety of cell types, including osteocytes, suggesting their effective use in bone regeneration, although clinical studies are limited. In addition to DPSCs and periosteal stem cells, adipose tissue also serves as a source of MSCs [17]. In fact, adipose-derived stromal cells can differentiate into chondrocytes, osteocytes, or myocytes, as indicated by several studies in animal models [54–57], although clear and conclusive data about their osteogenic potential are limited.

In 2005, Laino et al. [58] successfully isolated and selected a distinctive and highly enriched population of stem cells derived from dental pulp in adult humans. This stem cell population was self-expanding and differentiated into pre-osteoblasts able to self-maintain and renew. These stem cells differentiated into osteoblasts and produced living autologous fibrous bone tissue in vitro after 50 days of culture. Transplantation of this tissue in vivo led to the formation of lamellar bone with osteocytes without the need for scaffolding. The differentiated cells and living autologous fibrous bone could be frozen at −80°C and stored for extended periods of time with no clear effect on their bone-forming ability. The same research group subsequently demonstrated that DPSCs differentiate into osteoblasts that secrete abundant extracellular matrix [59].

In 2007, d'Aquino et al. [60] provided direct evidence that osteogenesis and angiogenesis mediated by human DPSCs are regulated by distinct mechanisms that lead to the organization of adult bone tissue after stem cell transplantation. In this study, stromal stem cells from human dental pulp were extracted, cultivated, and characterized in vitro. After 30 days of culture, the cells began to differentiate, lost their stem cell markers, and expressed differentiation markers. After 40 days, the cells differentiated into two cytotypes from a common progenitor: osteogenic progenitor cells (70% of total cells) and endothelial progenitor cells (EPCs, 30%), demonstrating synergic differentiation into osteoblasts and endotheliocytes. After 50 days, woven bone was obtained in vitro and its transplantation into immunocompromised rats resulted in a tissue structure with an integral blood supply similar to that of human adult bone. These findings suggest that osteogenesis and vasculogenesis are interdependent, and that this process is essential to obtain adult bone tissue suitable for transplantation and surgical or clinical applications in tissue repair.

DPSCs grafted into immunosuppressed rats generated complete and well-vascularized lamellar bone [61]. DPSCs are easily managed because they have a long lifespan, can be safely cryopreserved, and are able to interact with biomaterials [62]. Finally, in vitro and in vivo experiments revealed that both the quality and quantity of bone regenerated by DPSCs blended from stem cells and biomaterials [58, 60, 61, 63].

DPSCs can be applied for oral and maxillofacial bone repair in the maxillofacial area and, on appropriate resorbable scaffolds, promote the formation of an efficient biocomplex in patients with a mandibular defect, as reported by d'Aquino et al. [60]. In that study, a biocomplex constructed from dental pulp stem/progenitor cells and a collagen-sponge scaffold was used for oral and maxillofacial bone tissue repair. Stem/progenitor cells obtained from the upper third of molars previously extracted were gently placed with a syringe onto a collagen-sponge scaffold and used to fill the space left by the lower third of the molar extraction procedure. Thirty days after surgery, X-ray controls exhibited a high rate of mineralization; 3 months after the surgery, samples collected from the regeneration site showed well-organized and well-vascularized bone with a lamellar architecture surrounding the Haversian canals. Bone from control sites was immature and showed fibrous bone entrapped among new lamellae, incomplete and large Haversian canals, and evidence of bone resorption. Moreover, immu-nofluorescence analyses showed high levels of bone morphogenetic protein-2 and VEGF in regeneration samples. This clinical study demonstrated that dental pulp stem/progenitor cells can be used for oral and maxillofacial bone repair and that collagen sponges can be considered an optimal support for stem/progenitor cells in cell-guided regeneration.

The same group published a 3-year follow-up [64]. Histology and in-line holotomography revealed that regenerated bone was uniformly vascularized and qualitatively compact rather than the physiologic type of bone found in that region—cancellous (i.e., spongy). The authors speculated that the regeneration of compact bone probably occurs because grafted DPSCs do not follow the local signals of the surrounding spongy bone. Although the bone that regener-ated at the graft site was not the proper type found in the mandible, it seemed to have a positive clinical outcome because it created steadier mandibles, increased implant stability, and may have improved resistance to mechanical, physical, chemical, and pharmacologic agents.

Although the use of DPSCs is valid for tissue regeneration in the maxillofacial area, the identification of an accessible site from which to collect these cells can be challenging, and the amount of cells that can be obtained is very limited. DPSCs can be cultured by two methods. In the enzyme-digestion method, pulp tissue is collected under sterile conditions and digested with the appropriate enzymes, and the resulting cell suspensions are seeded in culture dishes [65]. In the explant outgrowth method, the extracted pulp tissues are cut, anchored via microcarriers onto a suitable substrate, and directly incubated in culture dishes [66]. From a clinical point of view, these methods are not appropriate for therapeutic applications because of the manipulation of dental pulp. A new, efficient, and safe method for isolating dental pulp was reported by Brunelli in 2013 [67], in which a new instrument called a Rigenera® (Torino, Italy) machine was used to create micrografts of disaggregated dental pulp that was subse-quently poured onto a collagen sponge. This micrograft was injected into the sinus cavity, and 4 months after the intervention newly formed bone was observed with twice the mineral density of native bone [67].

2.2. Periosteal stem cells

In addition to dental pulp, the periosteum is a surprising source of stem cells. After bone fracture in animal models, periosteal progenitor cells undergo an impressive expansion, followed by differentiation into osteoblasts and chondrocytes [68]. This remarkable property of the periosteum has prompted extensive research into the use of periosteum-derived cells for regenerative approaches, and preclinical studies have demonstrated the potential of these cells. The success of periosteal cells in preclinical animal models has also given rise to several exploratory clinical studies using ex vivo expanded periosteal cells for bone regeneration.

In 1992, chick tibial periosteal cells were cultured, combined with porous calcium phosphate ceramics, and subcutaneously implanted into athymic mice [69]. These cells eventually gave rise to bone tissue via two different mechanisms. Intramembranous bone formation occurred early in the peripheral pores of the ceramics, and endochondral bone formation occurred later in the central pores. These results raised the possibility that composite grafts of cultured periosteal-derived cells and porous ceramics could be clinically used as bone-graft substitutes for bone augmentation or regeneration.

In 2001, Vacanti et al. [70] first used culture-expanded periosteal cells derived from the radius in combination with a porous hydroxyapatite scaffold to replace the distal phalanx of the thumb. In this study, coral alone seeded with cells derived from the periosteum and placed in the subcutaneous tissue that was not adjacent to native bone formed new bone.

The use of periosteum-derived bony matrix for augmentation in the posterior maxilla before implantation results in bone formation 4 months after transplantation with trabecular bone containing viable osteocytes [71, 72]. The graft provides a reliable basis for the simultaneous or secondary insertion of dental implants.

Springer et al. [73] compared mandibular periosteum cells that were cultured and seeded onto a collagen matrix and maxillary bone cells that were cultured and seeded onto natural bone minerals. They concluded that the first method produced a significantly higher amount of new living bone.

Taken together, these reports demonstrate the clinical potential of periosteal-derived cells for bone regeneration therapies. The last three studies described, however, did not use stem cells but rather only cultures of differentiated periosteal cells.

2.3. Bone marrow-derived MSCs

Bone marrow-derived mesenchymal stem cells (BMSCs) are a readily available and abundant source of cells for tissue-engineering applications. BMSCs may be useful tools for regenerating bone, but the method of bone marrow aspiration from patients is associated with significant morbidity at the donor site [74].

BMSCs can differentiate into osteoblasts in vitro [75] and have osteogenic ability in vivo [76]. The addition of BMSCs to a biomaterial improves the quality of regenerated lamellar bone [77]. In 2008, BMSCs were successfully used in association with biphasic hydroxyapatite/β-tricalcium phosphate in a sinus-augmentation procedure [78].

In a recent study [79], tissue repair cells isolated from bone marrow were successfully used to repair bone defects in a human model. In this study, bone marrow cells were collected, cultivated, and characterized. Flow cytometry demonstrated the presence of mesenchymal and vascular phenotypes. The cellular suspension, carried by a gelatin sponge, was implanted in a postextraction site and covered by a resorbable collagen membrane. Six weeks after the implantation, biopsy revealed the presence of highly vascularized and mineralized bone tissue. McAllister et al. [5] used an MSC-heterologous bone graft harvested from cadavers for sinus-augmentation procedures. The authors demonstrated the presence of MSCs in the commercial bone preparation derived from cadavers and harvested within 24 h of death and stored at −80 °C. Moreover, they rapidly formed bone from a commercially available cellular bone matrix that contained heterologous MSCs.

In one study [80], researchers seeded Geistlich Bio-Oss (GeistlichPharma North America, Princeton, NJ, USA) with stem cells and found that this construct was superior to Bio-Oss mixed with autogenous bone in terms of bone formation 3–4 months after surgery. This study, however, presented some issues regarding data reporting and statistical analysis.

In a well-documented preliminary report, Behnia et al. [81] used BMSCs in association with platelet-rich plasma. They used biphasic hydroxyapatite/tricalcium phosphate as a scaffold and implanted the graft in an alveolar cleft, achieving cleft closure and a mean postoperative defect filling of 51.3% at 3 months after surgery. The same research group used demineralized bone mineral and calcium sulfate in association with BMSCs to treat alveolar clefts, but did not achieve similar positive results [47]. They concluded that the latter material was not a suitable scaffold for MSC-induced bone regeneration.

Bone marrow aspiration, however, is severely painful for donors, often requires general anesthesia, and may be associated with adverse events [74, 82].

2.4. Blood-derived stem cells

Peripheral blood is a source of MSCs that can be isolated with minimal invasiveness compared to extraction from bone marrow [83, 84]. According to some authors [85], blood-derived stem cells have characteristics and bone-regeneration abilities that are similar to those of BMSCs both in vitro and in vivo and are a promising source for bone regeneration for clinical use; by contrast, other authors [83] report that blood-derived stem cells have less multipotency than bone BMSCs.

2.5. Adipose-derived stem cells

Adipose tissue is an alternative source of MSCs that can differentiate into chondrocytes, osteocytes, or myocytes [17, 54, 86, 87]. An in vivo study demonstrated that adipose-derived stem cells are capable of bone regeneration and are useful for reconstructing critical-size defects in rats [55].

2.6. Secretomes

MSCs enhance wound healing, but the mechanisms are unclear. The use of MSCs for tissue repair was initially based on the hypothesis that these cells migrate to and differentiate within injured tissues, becoming specialized cells. It now appears that only a small proportion of transplanted MSCs actually integrate into and survive in the host tissue. Thus, the predominant mechanism by which MSCs participate in tissue repair seems to be related to their paracrine activity. Indeed, MSCs provide a suitable microenvironment that includes a multitude of trophic and survival signals, including growth factors and cytokines. Factors secreted from stem cells into a medium are called *secretomes* and have attracted much attention [45] because of their ability to support regenerative processes in the damaged tissue, induce angiogenesis, protect cells from apoptosis, modulate the immune system, and recruit endogenous stem cells to the grafted site. Compared to stem cells from other sources, BMSCs secrete distinctively different cytokines and chemokines, including greater amounts of VEGF-alpha, insulin-like growth factor 1, epidermal growth factor, keratinocyte growth factor, Ang-1, stromal-derived factor 1, macrophage inflammatory protein-1 alpha and -1 beta, and erythropoietin [45], which are important for normal wound healing.

In vitro, the CM from the culture of BMSCs (MSC-CM) enhances the migration, proliferation, and expression of osteogenic marker genes such as alkaline phosphatase, osteocalcin, and Runt-related transcription factor 2 of MSCs, and contains cytokines such as insulin-like growth factor 1, VEGF, transforming growth factor-β1, and hepatocyte growth factor. The concentrations of cytokines contained in MSC-CM are relatively low, and the use of MSC-CM does not induce the severe histologic inflammatory responses observed with the clinical use of recombinant human bone morphogenetic protein 2 [88]. Implantation of MSC-CM in association with a collagen sponge or agarose produced early bone regeneration in rat calvaria, suggesting that MSC-CM has potential for cell-free bone regeneration [88, 89].

MSC-CM recruits endogenous stem cells to the graft site and promotes early bone and periodontal regeneration in rat calvarial bone defects and periodontal tissue [88, 90]. Some authors [88] noted a stronger effect on bone regeneration and autogenous MSC migration when MSC-CM, rather than MSCs alone, was used in the graft, demonstrating that MSC-CM induces bone regeneration via mobilization of endogenous stem cells. The recent use of MSC-CM in various oral and maxillofacial bone regeneration procedures demonstrated osteogenic potential [91].

The use of MSC-CM for bone regeneration is a unique concept in which the paracrine factors of stem cells are used without cell transplantation.

3. Cell isolation

The isolation of cells is often difficult, and the methods of extraction, such as enzymatic digestion or mechanical disaggregation, require several minutes to a few hours, which can reduce cell viability. A recent study [92] demonstrated the efficacy of a new medical device called Rigeneracons® (CE certified Class I; Human Brain Wave, Turin, Italy) (**Figures 1** and **2**) to provide autologous periosteal micrografts (**Figure 3**) for clinical practice that are enriched with progenitor cells and are able to regenerate and differentiate.

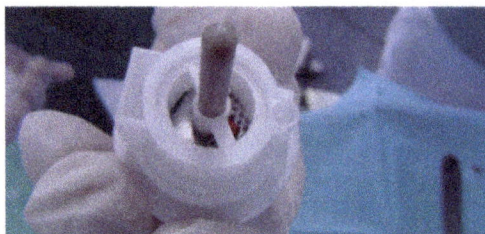

Figures 1. Rigeneracons® medical device.

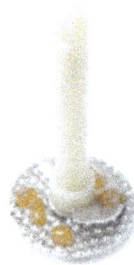

Figures 2. Detail of the blades system which disaggregate the periosteal tissue.

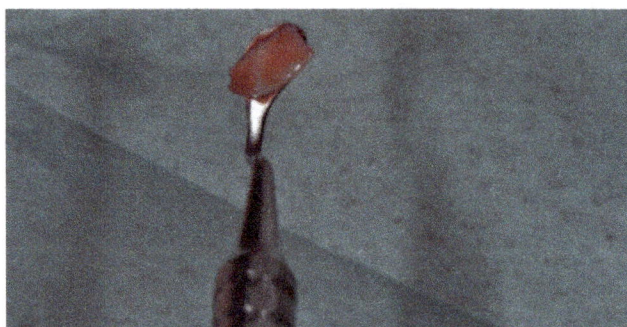

Figures 3. 1-2 mm² of periosteal tissue harvested after flap elevation can be disaggregate to get progenitor cells that will be seeded on a scaffold to be grafted in the bone defect.

The protocol is very simple. A 1–2-mm periosteal tissue harvested from the flap elevated at extraction or other surgical site is disaggregated mechanically (2 min at 15 Ncm and 75 round/min) after adding 1 ml sterile saline. The Rigeneracons® has 100 holes each provided with six microblades. A filter allows only the cells smaller than 50 μ (eight progenitor cells) to drop into a tank. The solution is then seeded on a polymeric scaffold (polylactic-co-glycolic acid-hydroxyapatite (PLGA-HA)) and grafted in the bone site (socket preservation, sinus lifting, periodontal defects, etc.) Although in vitro data about the Rigenera protocol are limited, a recent study demonstrated the efficacy of the Rigenera machine for obtaining stem cells from dental pulp [67]. These cells were positive for mesenchymal cell-line markers and negative for hematopoietic and macrophage markers. The percentage of viable cells derived from periosteum samples was high, however, suggesting that the device provides effective extraction.

4. Scaffold

MSCs grafted from a cell suspension require scaffolds to provide support, cohesion, and stability. Several types of materials are used as scaffolds. Advances in cell therapy have been accompanied by advances in novel scaffold fabrication techniques, yielding greater control over the surface topography, internal microstructure, and pore interconnectivity. Porous scaffolds have been widely explored for cell attachment because of the importance of allowing adequate room for tissue ingrowth and vascularization (i.e., pore size of 150–500 nm) [93]. Although natural materials retain their bioactivity, synthetic scaffolds present several advantages, including added flexibility in manufacturing, reproducibility, sterilization, storage times, and nonimmunogenicity. Solid free-form fabrication, a rapid three-dimensional printing technology for prototyping, was recently adapted for use in bone regeneration. Other researchers have developed hydrogels to encapsulate stem cells for tissue engineering, some with tunable degradation rates, but hydrogels may not provide the strength necessary for bone repair in load-bearing locations [94–96].

Not all researchers agree about the efficacy of combinations of stem cells and scaffolds, and a recent study reported that tissue-engineered complexes did not significantly improve bone-induced regeneration processes. Further studies are needed to elucidate the role of stem cells and scaffolds in tissue regeneration [97].

5. Epigenetic regulation

Epigenetic factors play a fundamental role in regulating the regenerative processes of MSCs [98, 99]. In stem cell differentiation processes, some genes may be upregulated and others repressed. Epigenetic modifications result in significant functional genomic alterations without changes in the nucleotide sequence [100].

Well-known epigenetic mechanisms include DNA methylation and histone modifications. Cytosine methylation downregulates gene expression, and the absence of methylation is essential for gene expression. In bone regeneration, however, methylation is essential. During MSC differentiation into osteoblasts in vitro, methylation of the osteocalcin promoter is significantly decreased, leading to the upregulation of osteocalcin [98]. Also, during osteoblast differentiation, increased methylation of the promoter of LIN28, a gene responsible for the maintenance of stem cell characteristics, reduces the expression of this gene, which facilitates osteogenesis [101].

Gene transcription is also regulated by histone modifications [100]. Histones are positively charged proteins that strongly bind the light-chain bearing structure of the double strand of phosphate-deoxyribose DNA. The binding of histone DNA determines the accessibility of transcription factors [102]. The most studied modifications are acetylation and methylation. Acetylation reduces DNA binding, allowing for greater gene expression. Conversely, deacetylation leads to a more compact chromatin structure, thus decreasing gene expression [103]. During differentiation, osteoblastic regions of the osteocalcin and osteocalcin promoters exhibit high levels of acetylation, which allows for greater accessibility of transcription factors. In addition, the downregulation of histone deacetylase-1 is an important process during osteogenesis [104]. These examples highlight the complexity of the effects of epigenetic regulation during bone regeneration.

6. Issues

Despite the initial success regarding the use of MSCs, some challenges remain as follows:

1. MSC removal requires invasive procedures that are associated with morbidity.

2. MSC proliferation and osteogenic differentiation potential decrease with age.

3. Inadequate vascular grafts of MSC carriers lead to cell death.

4. Difficulty accessing the repair site may limit the application of MSCs.

Recent studies revealed that implanted cells do not survive long [105]. One study showed a significant loss of cells within 24 h, and low numbers of transplanted cells survived at 12 weeks. Cells that did survive, however, underwent differentiation [106].

A crucial issue for autografts is cell viability; after collection, viability decreases to less than 50%, thereby reducing the regenerative capacities of the autografts. Cell death results from vessel interruption and subsequently reduced nutrition. Inadequate graft dimensions and tissue-size reductions to facilitate feeding can also lead to cell death. A promising approach to address this problem is the use of an instrument that preserves graft viability, such as by selecting small cells that are less susceptible to cell lysis.

Graft vascularization is a determining factor in cell survival, engraftment, and bone regeneration. In 1997, circulating EPCs were identified [107, 108]. EPCs participate in neovascularization processes [109], angiogenesis, vascular repair, restoration of blood flow after ischemia, distraction osteogenesis [110, 111], healing of fractures [111], and bone regeneration [112], and have an osteogenic potential. They are located mainly in the bone marrow and are mobilized as a result of biologic signals. The in vitro cultivation of mononuclear cell fractions under favorable conditions produces two EPC subtypes: early- and late-outgrowth endothelial cells [113]. Early-outgrowth endothelial cells survive less than 7 days in vitro, are characterized by a low rate of duplication, and induce transient angiogenesis principally for paracrine effects; late-outgrowth cells can expand to 100 cell population doublings, take root at the site of engraftment, and can differentiate into osteoblasts [114]. A 2009 study demonstrated the successful application of blood-derived EPCs for healing bone defects [115].

7. Safety of transplanted MSCs

Clinical trials to evaluate the safety of MSCs for the treatment of graft-versus-host disease, ischemic heart disease, spinal cord injury, and systemic lupus erythematosus have not revealed any significant adverse effects [116–119]. While pluripotent cells have been obtained from adult somatic tissues by reprogramming methods [120], these cells can differentiate into different tissues and have wrongly been considered a source of MSCs for tissue regeneration. Indeed, they are known to cause teratoma formation and significant efforts to address the safety concerns are required before their application in patients [120]. By contrast, MSCs obtained without genetic reprogramming have a high capability to differentiate into many tissues without developing into tumor cells.

Studies of the role of MSCs in tumorigenesis have identified the ability of MSCs to interact with tumor cells and to support angiogenesis by providing a matrix to support cancer cells [121, 122]. MSCs may thus facilitate the growth of existing tumors [123, 124]. Transdifferentiation of MSCs has been observed in vitro, but this phenomenon could be due to contamination by tumor cells [125, 126].

Author details

Ruggero Rodriguez y Baena*, Silvana Rizzo, Antonio Graziano and Saturnino Marco Lupi

*Address all correspondence to: ruggero.rodriguez@unipv.it

Department of Clinico Surgical, Diagnostic and Pediatric Sciences, School of Dentistry, University of Pavia, Pavia, Italy

References

[1] Glimcher MJ. The nature of the mineral component of bone and the mechanism of calcification. Instructional Course Lectures. 1987;36:49–69.

[2] Buckwalter JA, Cooper RR. Bone structure and function. Instructional Course Lectures. 1987;36:27–48.

[3] Lanyon LE. Osteocytes, strain detection, bone modeling and remodeling. Calcified Tissue International. 1993;53 Suppl 1:S102–6; discussion S6–7.

[4] Roodman GD. Advances in bone biology: the osteoclast. Endocrine Reviews. 1996;17(4):308–32.

[5] McAllister BS, Haghighat K, Gonshor A. Histologic evaluation of a stem cell-based sinus-augmentation procedure. Journal of Periodontology. 2009;80(4):679–86.

[6] Caplan AI. Mesenchymal stem cells. Journal of Orthopaedic Research: Official Publication of the Orthopaedic Research Society. 1991;9(5):641–50.

[7] Caplan AI. The mesengenic process. Clinics in Plastic Surgery. 1994;21(3):429–35.

[8] Caplan AI. Review: mesenchymal stem cells: cell-based reconstructive therapy in orthopedics. Tissue Engineering. 2005;11(7–8):1198–211.

[9] Friedenstein AJ, Petrakova KV, Kurolesova AI, Frolova GP. Heterotopic of bone marrow. Analysis of precursor cells for osteogenic and hematopoietic tissues. Transplantation. 1968;6(2):230–47.

[10] Fridenshtein A, Piatetskii S, II, Petrakova KV. Osteogenesis in transplants of bone 26 marrow cells. Arkhiv anatomii, gistologii i embriologii. 1969;56(3):3–11.

[11] Shanti RM, Li WJ, Nesti LJ, Wang X, Tuan RS. Adult mesenchymal stem cells: biological properties, characteristics, and applications in maxillofacial surgery. Journal of Oral and Maxillofacial Surgery: Official Journal of the American Association of Oral and Maxillofacial Surgeons. 2007;65(8):1640–7.

[12] Dominici M, Le Blanc K, Mueller I, Slaper-Cortenbach I, Marini F, Krause D, et al. Minimal criteria for defining multipotent mesenchymal stromal cells. The International Society for Cellular Therapy position statement. Cytotherapy. 2006;8(4):315–7.

[13] Barry FP, Murphy JM. Mesenchymal stem cells: clinical applications and biological characterization. The International Journal of Biochemistry & Cell Biology. 2004;36(4): 568–84.

[14] Sharma RR, Pollock K, Hubel A, McKenna D. Mesenchymal stem or stromal cells: a review of clinical applications and manufacturing practices. Transfusion. 2014;54(5): 1418–37.

[15] Pittenger MF, Mackay AM, Beck SC, Jaiswal RK, Douglas R, Mosca JD, et al. Multilineage potential of adult human mesenchymal stem cells. Science. 1999;284(5411):143–7.

[16] Erices A, Conget P, Minguell JJ. Mesenchymal progenitor cells in human umbilical cord blood. British Journal of Haematology. 2000;109(1):235–42.

[17] Zuk PA, Zhu M, Ashjian P, De Ugarte DA, Huang JI, Mizuno H, et al. Human adipose tissue is a source of multipotent stem cells. Molecular Biology of the cell. 2002;13(12): 4279–95.

[18] Jankowski RJ, Deasy BM, Huard J. Muscle-derived stem cells. Gene Therapy. 2002;9(10):642–7.

[19] Fukumoto T, Sperling JW, Sanyal A, Fitzsimmons JS, Reinholz GG, Conover CA, et al. Combined effects of insulin-like growth factor-1 and transforming growth factor-beta1 on periosteal mesenchymal cells during chondrogenesis in vitro. Osteoarthritis and Cartilage/OARS, Osteoarthritis Research Society. 2003;11(1):55–64.

[20] De Bari C, Dell'Accio F, Tylzanowski P, Luyten FP. Multipotent mesenchymal stem cells from adult human synovial membrane. Arthritis and Rheumatism. 2001;44(8): 1928–42.

[21] Miura M, Gronthos S, Zhao M, Lu B, Fisher LW, Robey PG, et al. SHED: stem cells from human exfoliated deciduous teeth. Proceedings of the National Academy of Sciences of the United States of America. 2003;100(10):5807–12.

[22] Crisan M, Yap S, Casteilla L, Chen CW, Corselli M, Park TS, et al. A perivascular origin for mesenchymal stem cells in multiple human organs. Cell Stem Cell. 2008;3(3):301– 13.

[23] Deschaseaux F, Pontikoglou C, Sensebe L. Bone regeneration: the stem/progenitor cells point of view. Journal of Cellular and Molecular Medicine. 2010;14(1–2):103–15.

[24] Paul G, Ozen I, Christophersen NS, Reinbothe T, Bengzon J, Visse E, et al. The adult human brain harbors multipotent perivascular mesenchymal stem cells. PLoS One. 2012;7(4):e35577.

[25] Miura M, Miura Y, Sonoyama W, Yamaza T, Gronthos S, Shi S. Bone marrow-derived mesenchymal stem cells for regenerative medicine in craniofacial region. Oral Diseases. 2006;12(6):514–22.

[26] Horwitz EM, Prockop DJ, Fitzpatrick LA, Koo WW, Gordon PL, Neel M, et al. Trans-plantability and therapeutic effects of bone marrow-derived mesenchymal cells in children with osteogenesis imperfecta. Nature Medicine. 1999;5(3):309–13.

[27] Petite H, Viateau V, Bensaid W, Meunier A, de Pollak C, Bourguignon M, et al. Tissue-engineered bone regeneration. Nature Biotechnology. 2000;18(9):959–63.

[28] Bruder SP, Kraus KH, Goldberg VM, Kadiyala S. The effect of implants loaded with autologous mesenchymal stem cells on the healing of canine segmental bone defects. The Journal of Bone and Joint Surgery American Volume. 1998;80(7):985–96.

[29] Zigdon-Giladi H, Bick T, Lewinson D, Machtei EE. Mesenchymal stem cells and endothelial progenitor cells stimulate bone regeneration and mineral density. Journal of Periodontology. 2014;85(7):984–90.

[30] Czerwinski M, Hopper RA, Gruss J, Fearon JA. Major morbidity and mortality rates in craniofacial surgery: an analysis of 8101 major procedures. Plastic and Reconstructive Surgery. 2010;126(1):181–6.

[31] Neovius E, Engstrand T. Craniofacial reconstruction with bone and biomaterials: review over the last 11 years. Journal of Plastic, Reconstructive & Aesthetic Surgery: JPRAS. 2010;63(10):1615–23.

[32] Hollinger JO, Winn S, Bonadio J. Options for tissue engineering to address challenges of the aging skeleton. Tissue Engineering. 2000;6(4):341–50.

[33] Korbling M, Estrov Z. Adult stem cells for tissue repair – a new therapeutic concept? The New England Journal of Medicine. 2003;349(6):570–82.

[34] Tolar J, Le Blanc K, Keating A, Blazar BR. Concise review: hitting the right spot with mesenchymal stromal cells. Stem Cells. 2010;28(8):1446–55.

[35] Blau HM, Brazelton TR, Weimann JM. The evolving concept of a stem cell: entity or function? Cell. 2001;105(7):829–41.

[36] Gnecchi M, Zhang Z, Ni A, Dzau VJ. Paracrine mechanisms in adult stem cell signaling and therapy. Circulation Research. 2008;103(11):1204–19.

[37] Phinney DG. Biochemical heterogeneity of mesenchymal stem cell populations: clues to their therapeutic efficacy. Cell Cycle. 2007;6(23):2884–9.

[38] Meirelles Lda S, Fontes AM, Covas DT, Caplan AI. Mechanisms involved in the therapeutic properties of mesenchymal stem cells. Cytokine & Growth Factor Reviews. 2009;20(5–6):419–27.

[39] Hocking AM, Gibran NS. Mesenchymal stem cells: paracrine signaling and differentiation during cutaneous wound repair. Experimental Cell Research. 2010;316(14): 2213–9.

[40] Maltman DJ, Hardy SA, Przyborski SA. Role of mesenchymal stem cells in neurogenesis and nervous system repair. Neurochemistry International. 2011;59(3):347–56.

[41] Ankrum J, Karp JM. Mesenchymal stem cell therapy: two steps forward, one step back. Trends in Molecular Medicine. 2010;16(5):203–9.

[42] Horie M, Choi H, Lee RH, Reger RL, Ylostalo J, Muneta T, et al. Intra-articular injection of human mesenchymal stem cells (MSCs) promote rat meniscal regeneration by being activated to express Indian hedgehog that enhances expression of type II collagen. Osteoarthritis and Cartilage/OARS, Osteoarthritis Research Society. 2012;20(10):1197–207.

[43] Mirotsou M, Jayawardena TM, Schmeckpeper J, Gnecchi M, Dzau VJ. Paracrine mechanisms of stem cell reparative and regenerative actions in the heart. Journal of Molecular and Cellular Cardiology. 2011;50(2):280–9.

[44] Walter MN, Wright KT, Fuller HR, MacNeil S, Johnson WE. Mesenchymal stem cell-conditioned medium accelerates skin wound healing: an in vitro study of fibroblast and keratinocyte scratch assays. Experimental Cell Research. 2010;316(7):1271–81.

[45] Chen L, Tredget EE, Wu PY, Wu Y. Paracrine factors of mesenchymal stem cells recruit macrophages and endothelial lineage cells and enhance wound healing. PLoS One. 2008;3(4):e1886.

[46] Horn AP, Frozza RL, Grudzinski PB, Gerhardt D, Hoppe JB, Bruno AN, et al. Conditioned medium from mesenchymal stem cells induces cell death in organotypic cultures of rat hippocampus and aggravates lesion in a model of oxygen and glucose deprivation. Neuroscience Research. 2009;63(1):35–41.

[47] Behnia H, Khojasteh A, Soleimani M, Tehranchi A, Khoshzaban A, Keshel SH, et al. Secondary repair of alveolar clefts using human mesenchymal stem cells. Oral surgery, Oral Medicine, Oral Pathology, Oral Radiology, and Endodontics. 2009;108(2):e1–6.

[48] Park JB. Use of cell-based approaches in maxillary sinus augmentation procedures. The Journal of Craniofacial Surgery. 2010;21(2):557–60.

[49] Caplan AI. New era of cell-based orthopedic therapies. Tissue Engineering Part B, Reviews. 2009;15(2):195–200.

[50] Steinhardt Y, Aslan H, Regev E, Zilberman Y, Kallai I, Gazit D, et al. Maxillofacial-derived stem cells regenerate critical mandibular bone defect. Tissue Engineering Part A. 2008;14(11):1763–73.

[51] Ben-David D, Kizhner TA, Kohler T, Muller R, Livne E, Srouji S. Cell-scaffold transplant of hydrogel seeded with rat bone marrow progenitors for bone regeneration. Journal of Cranio-maxillo-facial Surgery: Official Publication of the European Association for Cranio-Maxillo-Facial Surgery. 2011;39(5):364–71.

[52] Jo YY, Lee HJ, Kook SY, Choung HW, Park JY, Chung JH, et al. Isolation and characterization of postnatal stem cells from human dental tissues. Tissue Engineering. 2007;13(4):767–73.

[53] Lensch MW, Daheron L, Schlaeger TM. Pluripotent stem cells and their niches. Stem Cell Reviews. 2006;2(3):185–201.

[54] Levi B, Longaker MT. Concise review: adipose-derived stromal cells for skeletal regenerative medicine. Stem Cells. 2011;29(4):576–82.

[55] Streckbein P, Jackel S, Malik CY, Obert M, Kahling C, Wilbrand JF, et al. Reconstruction of critical-size mandibular defects in immunoincompetent rats with human adipose-derived stromal cells. Journal of Cranio-maxillo-facial Surgery: Official Publication of the European Association for Cranio-Maxillo-Facial Surgery. 2013;41(6):496–503.

[56] Linero I, Chaparro O. Paracrine effect of mesenchymal stem cells derived from human adipose tissue in bone regeneration. PLoS One. 2014;9(9):e107001.

[57] Stromps JP, Paul NE, Rath B, Nourbakhsh M, Bernhagen J, Pallua N. Chondrogenic differentiation of human adipose-derived stem cells: a new path in articular cartilage defect management? BioMed Research International. 2014;2014:740926.

[58] Laino G, d'Aquino R, Graziano A, Lanza V, Carinci F, Naro F, et al. A new population of human adult dental pulp stem cells: a useful source of living autologous fibrous bone tissue (LAB). Journal of Bone and Mineral Research: the Official Journal of the American Society for Bone and Mineral Research. 2005;20(8):1394–402.

[59] Laino G, Carinci F, Graziano A, d'Aquino R, Lanza V, De Rosa A, et al. In vitro bone production using stem cells derived from human dental pulp. The Journal of Craniofacial Surgery. 2006;17(3):511–5.

[60] d'Aquino R, Graziano A, Sampaolesi M, Laino G, Pirozzi G, De Rosa A, et al. Human postnatal dental pulp cells co-differentiate into osteoblasts and endotheliocytes: a pivotal synergy leading to adult bone tissue formation. Cell Death and Differentiation. 2007;14(6):1162–71.

[61] Graziano A, d'Aquino R, Cusella-De Angelis MG, De Francesco F, Giordano A, Laino G, et al. Scaffold's surface geometry significantly affects human stem cell bone tissue engineering. Journal of Cellular Physiology. 2008;214(1):166–72.

[62] Papaccio G, Graziano A, d'Aquino R, Graziano MF, Pirozzi G, Menditti D, et al. Long-term cryopreservation of dental pulp stem cells (SBP-DPSCs) and their differentiated osteoblasts: a cell source for tissue repair. Journal of cellular physiology. 2006;208(2):319–25.

[63] Graziano A, d'Aquino R, Laino G, Papaccio G. Dental pulp stem cells: a promising tool for bone regeneration. Stem Cell Reviews. 2008;4(1):21–6.

[64] Giuliani A, Manescu A, Langer M, Rustichelli F, Desiderio V, Paino F, et al. Three years after transplants in human mandibles, histological and in-line holotomography revealed that stem cells regenerated a compact rather than a spongy bone: biological and clinical implications. Stem Cells Translational Medicine. 2013;2(4):316–24.

[65] Sonoyama W, Liu Y, Yamaza T, Tuan RS, Wang S, Shi S, et al. Characterization of the apical papilla and its residing stem cells from human immature permanent teeth: a pilot study. Journal of Endodontics. 2008;34(2):166–71.

[66] Saito T, Ogawa M, Hata Y, Bessho K. Acceleration effect of human recombinant bone morphogenetic protein-2 on differentiation of human pulp cells into odontoblasts. Journal of Endodontics. 2004;30(4):205–8.

[67] Brunelli G, Motroni A, Graziano A, D'Aquino R, Zollino I, Carinci F. Sinus lift tissue engineering using autologous pulp micro-grafts: a case report of bone density evaluation. Journal of Indian Society of Periodontology. 2013;17(5):644–7.

[68] Colnot C. Skeletal cell fate decisions within periosteum and bone marrow during bone regeneration. Journal of Bone and Mineral Research: the Official Journal of the American Society for Bone and Mineral Research. 2009;24(2):274–82.

[69] Nakahara H, Goldberg VM, Caplan AI. Culture-expanded periosteal-derived cells exhibit osteochondrogenic potential in porous calcium phosphate ceramics in vivo. Clinical Orthopaedics and Related Research. 1992(276):291–8.

[70] Vacanti CA, Bonassar LJ, Vacanti MP, Shufflebarger J. Replacement of an avulsed phalanx with tissue-engineered bone. The New England Journal of Medicine. 2001;344(20):1511–4.

[71] Schimming R, Schmelzeisen R. Tissue-engineered bone for maxillary sinus augmentation. Journal of Oral and Maxillofacial Surgery: Official Journal of the American Association of Oral and Maxillofacial Surgeons. 2004;62(6):724–9.

[72] Schmelzeisen R, Schimming R, Sittinger M. Making bone: implant insertion into tissue-engineered bone for maxillary sinus floor augmentation-a preliminary report. Journal of Cranio-maxillo-facial surgery: Official Publication of the European Association for Cranio-Maxillo-Facial Surgery. 2003;31(1):34–9.

[73] Springer IN, Nocini PF, Schlegel KA, De Santis D, Park J, Warnke PH, et al. Two techniques for the preparation of cell-scaffold constructs suitable for sinus augmentation: steps into clinical application. Tissue Engineering. 2006;12(9):2649–56.

[74] Bain BJ. Bone marrow biopsy morbidity: review of 2003. Journal of Clinical Pathology. 2005;58(4):406–8.

[75] Ogura N, Kawada M, Chang WJ, Zhang Q, Lee SY, Kondoh T, et al. Differentiation of the human mesenchymal stem cells derived from bone marrow and enhancement of cell attachment by fibronectin. Journal of Oral Science. 2004;46(4):207–13.

[76] Dong J, Kojima H, Uemura T, Kikuchi M, Tateishi T, Tanaka J. In vivo evaluation of a novel porous hydroxyapatite to sustain osteogenesis of transplanted bone marrow-derived osteoblastic cells. Journal of Biomedical Materials Research. 2001;57(2):208–16.

[77] Jafarian M, Eslaminejad MB, Khojasteh A, Mashhadi Abbas F, Dehghan MM, Hassanizadeh R, et al. Marrow-derived mesenchymal stem cells-directed bone regeneration in the dog mandible: a comparison between biphasic calcium phosphate and natural bone mineral. Oral Surgery, Oral Medicine, Oral Pathology, Oral Radiology, and Endodontics. 2008;105(5):e14–24.

[78] Shayesteh YS, Khojasteh A, Soleimani M, Alikhasi M, Khoshzaban A, Ahmadbeigi N. Sinus augmentation using human mesenchymal stem cells loaded into a beta-tricalcium phosphate/hydroxyapatite scaffold. Oral Surgery, Oral Medicine, Oral Pathology, Oral Radiology, and Endodontics. 2008;106(2):203–9.

[79] Kaigler D, Pagni G, Park CH, Braun TM, Holman LA, Yi E, et al. Stem cell therapy for craniofacial bone regeneration: a randomized, controlled feasibility trial. Cell Transplantation. 2013;22(5):767–77.

[80] Rickert D, Sauerbier S, Nagursky H, Menne D, Vissink A, Raghoebar GM. Maxillary sinus floor elevation with bovine bone mineral combined with either autogenous bone

or autogenous stem cells: a prospective randomized clinical trial. Clinical Oral Implants Research. 2011;22(3):251–8.

[81] Behnia H, Khojasteh A, Soleimani M, Tehranchi A, Atashi A. Repair of alveolar cleft defect with mesenchymal stem cells and platelet derived growth factors: a preliminary report. Journal of Cranio-maxillo-facial surgery: Official Publication of the European Association for Cranio-Maxillo-Facial Surgery. 2012;40(1):2–7.

[82] Mizuno H, Hyakusoku H. Mesengenic potential and future clinical perspective of human processed lipoaspirate cells. Journal of Nippon Medical School = Nippon Ika Daigaku zasshi. 2003;70(4):300–6.

[83] Koerner J, Nesic D, Romero JD, Brehm W, Mainil-Varlet P, Grogan SP. Equine peripheral blood-derived progenitors in comparison to bone marrow-derived mesenchymal stem cells. Stem Cells. 2006;24(6):1613–9.

[84] Zvaifler NJ, Marinova-Mutafchieva L, Adams G, Edwards CJ, Moss J, Burger JA, et al. Mesenchymal precursor cells in the blood of normal individuals. Arthritis Research. 2000;2(6):477–88.

[85] Zheng RC, Park YK, Kim SK, Cho J, Heo SJ, Koak JY, et al. Bone regeneration of blood-derived stem cells within dental implants. Journal of Dental Research. 2015;94(9):1318–25.

[86] Dragoo JL, Choi JY, Lieberman JR, Huang J, Zuk PA, Zhang J, et al. Bone induction by BMP-2 transduced stem cells derived from human fat. Journal of Orthopaedic Research: Official Publication of the Orthopaedic Research Society. 2003;21(4):622–9.

[87] Lee JA, Parrett BM, Conejero JA, Laser J, Chen J, Kogon AJ, et al. Biological alchemy: engineering bone and fat from fat-derived stem cells. Annals of Plastic Surgery. 2003;50(6):610–7.

[88] Osugi M, Katagiri W, Yoshimi R, Inukai T, Hibi H, Ueda M. Conditioned media from mesenchymal stem cells enhanced bone regeneration in rat calvarial bone defects. Tissue Engineering Part A. 2012;18(13–14):1479–89.

[89] Katagiri W, Osugi M, Kawai T, Ueda M. Novel cell-free regeneration of bone using stem cell-derived growth factors. The International Journal of Oral & Maxillofacial Implants. 2013;28(4):1009–16.

[90] Kawai T, Katagiri W, Osugi M, Sugimura Y, Hibi H, Ueda M. Secretomes from bone marrow-derived mesenchymal stromal cells enhance periodontal tissue regeneration. Cytotherapy. 2015;17(4):369–81.

[91] Katagiri W, Osugi M, Kawai T, Hibi H. First-in-human study and clinical case reports of the alveolar bone regeneration with the secretome from human mesenchymal stem cells. Head & Face Medicine. 2016;12(1):5.

[92] Trovato L, Monti M, Del Fante C, Cervio M, Lampinen M, Ambrosio L, et al. A new medical device rigeneracons allows to obtain viable micro-grafts from mechanical

disaggregation of human tissues. Journal of Cellular Physiology. 2015;230(10):2299–303.

[93] Scaglione S, Giannoni P, Bianchini P, Sandri M, Marotta R, Firpo G, et al. Order versus disorder: in vivo bone formation within osteoconductive scaffolds. Scientific Reports. 2012;2:274.

[94] Park H, Temenoff JS, Tabata Y, Caplan AI, Mikos AG. Injectable biodegradable hydrogel composites for rabbit marrow mesenchymal stem cell and growth factor delivery for cartilage tissue engineering. Biomaterials. 2007;28(21):3217–27.

[95] Alsberg E, Anderson KW, Albeiruti A, Franceschi RT, Mooney DJ. Cell-interactive alginate hydrogels for bone tissue engineering. Journal of Dental Research. 2001;80(11): 2025–9.

[96] Betz MW, Modi PC, Caccamese JF, Coletti DP, Sauk JJ, Fisher JP. Cyclic acetal hydrogel system for bone marrow stromal cell encapsulation and osteodifferentiation. Journal of Biomedical Materials Research Part A. 2008;86(3):662–70.

[97] Annibali S, Cicconetti A, Cristalli MP, Giordano G, Trisi P, Pilloni A, et al. A comparative morphometric analysis of biodegradable scaffolds as carriers for dental pulp and periosteal stem cells in a model of bone regeneration. The Journal of Craniofacial Surgery. 2013;24(3):866–71.

[98] Villagra A, Gutierrez J, Paredes R, Sierra J, Puchi M, Imschenetzky M, et al. Reduced CpG methylation is associated with transcriptional activation of the bone-specific rat osteocalcin gene in osteoblasts. Journal of Cellular Biochemistry. 2002;85(1):112–22.

[99] Arnsdorf EJ, Tummala P, Castillo AB, Zhang F, Jacobs CR. The epigenetic mechanism of mechanically induced osteogenic differentiation. Journal of Biomechanics. 2010;43(15):2881–6.

[100] Jaenisch R, Bird A. Epigenetic regulation of gene expression: how the genome integrates intrinsic and environmental signals. Nature Genetics. 2003;33 Suppl:245–54.

[101] Dansranjavin T, Krehl S, Mueller T, Mueller LP, Schmoll HJ, Dammann RH. The role of promoter CpG methylation in the epigenetic control of stem cell related genes during differentiation. Cell Cycle. 2009;8(6):916–24.

[102] Zheng C, Hayes JJ. Structures and interactions of the core histone tail domains. Biopolymers. 2003;68(4):539–46.

[103] Kouzarides T. Chromatin modifications and their function. Cell. 2007;128(4):693–705.

[104] Lee HW, Suh JH, Kim AY, Lee YS, Park SY, Kim JB. Histone deacetylase 1-mediated histone modification regulates osteoblast differentiation. Molecular Endocrinology. 2006;20(10):2432–43.

[105] Toma C, Wagner WR, Bowry S, Schwartz A, Villanueva F. Fate of culture-expanded mesenchymal stem cells in the microvasculature: in vivo observations of cell kinetics. Circulation Research. 2009;104(3):398–402.

[106] Muller-Ehmsen J, Whittaker P, Kloner RA, Dow JS, Sakoda T, Long TI, et al. Survival and development of neonatal rat cardiomyocytes transplanted into adult myocardium. Journal of Molecular and Cellular Cardiology. 2002;34(2):107–16.

[107] Asahara T, Murohara T, Sullivan A, Silver M, van der Zee R, Li T, et al. Isolation of putative progenitor endothelial cells for angiogenesis. Science. 1997;275(5302):964–7.

[108] Murohara T, Ikeda H, Duan J, Shintani S, Sasaki K, Eguchi H, et al. Transplanted cord blood-derived endothelial precursor cells augment postnatal neovascularization. The Journal of Clinical Investigation. 2000;105(11):1527–36.

[109] Takahashi T, Kalka C, Masuda H, Chen D, Silver M, Kearney M, et al. Ischemia- and cytokine-induced mobilization of bone marrow-derived endothelial progenitor cells for neovascularization. Nature Medicine. 1999;5(4):434–8.

[110] Lee DY, Cho TJ, Lee HR, Park MS, Yoo WJ, Chung CY, et al. Distraction osteogenesis induces endothelial progenitor cell mobilization without inflammatory response in man. Bone. 2010;46(3):673–9.

[111] Cetrulo CL, Jr., Knox KR, Brown DJ, Ashinoff RL, Dobryansky M, Ceradini DJ, et al. Stem cells and distraction osteogenesis: endothelial progenitor cells home to the ischemic generate in activation and consolidation. Plastic and Reconstructive Surgery. 2005;116(4):1053–64; discussion 65–7.

[112] Seebach C, Henrich D, Kahling C, Wilhelm K, Tami AE, Alini M, et al. Endothelial progenitor cells and mesenchymal stem cells seeded onto beta-TCP granules enhance early vascularization and bone healing in a critical-sized bone defect in rats. Tissue Engineering Part A. 2010;16(6):1961–70.

[113] Hur J, Yoon CH, Kim HS, Choi JH, Kang HJ, Hwang KK, et al. Characterization of two types of endothelial progenitor cells and their different contributions to neovasculo-genesis. Arteriosclerosis, Thrombosis, and Vascular Biology. 2004;24(2):288–93.

[114] Goligorsky MS, Salven P. Concise review: endothelial stem and progenitor cells and their habitats. Stem Cells Translational Medicine. 2013;2(7):499–504.

[115] Rozen N, Bick T, Bajayo A, Shamian B, Schrift-Tzadok M, Gabet Y, et al. Transplanted blood-derived endothelial progenitor cells (EPC) enhance bridging of sheep tibia critical size defects. Bone. 2009;45(5):918–24.

[116] Battiwalla M, Hematti P. Mesenchymal stem cells in hematopoietic stem cell transplantation. Cytotherapy. 2009;11(5):503–15.

[117] Lucchini G, Introna M, Dander E, Rovelli A, Balduzzi A, Bonanomi S, et al. Platelet-lysate-expanded mesenchymal stromal cells as a salvage therapy for severe resistant graft-versus-host disease in a pediatric population. Biology of Blood and Marrow

Transplantation: Journal of the American Society for Blood and Marrow Transplantation. 2010;16(9):1293–301.

[118] Pal R, Venkataramana NK, Bansal A, Balaraju S, Jan M, Chandra R, et al. Ex vivo-expanded autologous bone marrow-derived mesenchymal stromal cells in human spinal cord injury/paraplegia: a pilot clinical study. Cytotherapy. 2009;11(7):897–911.

[119] Sun L, Akiyama K, Zhang H, Yamaza T, Hou Y, Zhao S, et al. Mesenchymal stem cell transplantation reverses multiorgan dysfunction in systemic lupus erythematosus mice and humans. Stem Cells. 2009;27(6):1421–32.

[120] Hong SG, Winkler T, Wu C, Guo V, Pittaluga S, Nicolae A, et al. Path to the clinic: assessment of iPSC-based cell therapies in vivo in a nonhuman primate model. Cell Reports. 2014;7(4):1298–309.

[121] Ahn GO, Brown JM. Role of endothelial progenitors and other bone marrow-derived cells in the development of the tumor vasculature. Angiogenesis. 2009;12(2):159–64.

[122] Zhu W, Xu W, Jiang R, Qian H, Chen M, Hu J, et al. Mesenchymal stem cells derived from bone marrow favor tumor cell growth in vivo. Experimental and Molecular Pathology. 2006;80(3):267–74.

[123] Feng B, Chen L. Review of mesenchymal stem cells and tumors: executioner or coconspirator? Cancer Biotherapy & Radiopharmaceuticals. 2009;24(6):717–21.

[124] Motaln H, Schichor C, Lah TT. Human mesenchymal stem cells and their use in cell-based therapies. Cancer. 2010;116(11):2519–30.

[125] Garcia S, Bernad A, Martin MC, Cigudosa JC, Garcia-Castro J, de la Fuente R. Pitfalls in spontaneous in vitro transformation of human mesenchymal stem cells. Experimental Cell Research. 2010;316(9):1648–50.

[126] Torsvik A, Rosland GV, Svendsen A, Molven A, Immervoll H, McCormack E, et al. Spontaneous malignant transformation of human mesenchymal stem cells reflects cross-contamination: putting the research field on track – letter. Cancer Research. 2010;70(15):6393–6.

4

Use of Intra-Oral Osmotic Self-Inflating Tissue Expanders for Bone Reconstruction and Rehabilitation of the Jaws

Farzin Sarkarat, Farshid Kavandi,
Rouzbeh Kahali and
Mohammad Hosein Kalantar Motamedi

Abstract

Reconstruction of oral and maxillofacial defects is challenging. Insufficient soft tissues may render hard tissue reconstruction problematic. Several surgical techniques have been used over time to address this issue; these techniques are usually complicated and unpredictable. Soft tissue expansion is a physiological process that leads to the formation of new cells and growth of tissue and allows for soft tissue with similar color, texture and function to that of the adjacent tissues. In this article we present the applications of osmotic tissue expanders in facilitating bone graft augmentation. OSMED (Ilmenau, Germany) self-inflating tissue expanders were used prior to bone augmentation in our patients. After making a 1.5 cm full thickness incision, a sub-periosteal tunnel was prepared and the tissue expander was implanted sub-periosteally. The tissue expanders were removed approximately 6–10 weeks later in the course of augmentation surgery. In all patients after the use of the tissue expander, sufficient soft tissue was available for primary, tension-free, wound closure and there was no need for local or regional flap techniques. No complications such as infection, necrosis, or graft loss occurred and the functional and esthetic outcomes were acceptable. Use of this tissue expander prior to bone augmentation was effective in facilitating bone graft augmentation.

Keywords: Soft tissue expander, bone augmentation, reconstruction, soft tissue management, osmotic-tissue expanders

1. Introduction

Reconstruction of oral and maxillofacial defects is challenging. These defects may be congenital malformations, defects caused by severe atrophy, trauma or oncologic ablation. Such cases can cause considerable esthetics and/or functional problems and may require augmentation, grafting, and implantation procedures that may significantly affect the quality of life of the patients [1].

Insufficient hard and soft tissues may present esthetics or functional problems. Bone grafts, bone substitutes and guided tissue regeneration (GTR) techniques have been used for many years to rebuild the alveolar ridge [2]. Reconstructing large and complex defects are more complicated. One of the common problems is inadequate soft tissue for coverage of the graft. Several surgical techniques such as rotational flaps, pedicle flaps, free flaps and composite flaps have been used over time to address this issue [3, 4]; these techniques are usually complicated and they have limitations, such as donor site morbidity, necrosis and infection [4]. Another problem is the unpleasant functional and esthetics results due to the differences of the grafted tissues from the original tissue. One of the most common problems during reconstruction of bony defects of the jaws is soft tissue dehiscence which leads to the exposure of the bone grafts into the oral cavity and may result in loss of the bone graft [5–9]. Adequate soft tissue coverage of grafted bone is important to avoid graft exposure; thus, primary tension-free closure of the flap without compromising the vascularization is important [10–12]. When a large amount of bone augmentation is required, it is usually hard to achieve tension free soft tissue coverage. A periosteal incision is often used to make it possible to mobilize and stretch the mucoperiosteal flap. This, however, reduces the perfusion of the mucoperiosteal flap [11, 13–16]. Sufficient blood flow is important for tissue survival [17]. Even simple flap elevation can disturb flap perfusion and causes ischemia [18]. Extensive flap preparation and elevation can result in impaired perfusion and increased incidence of necrosis and tissue dehiscence [19, 20]. Inadequate perfusion and dehiscence of the soft tissue can jeopardize the success of bone augmentation.

One possible solution is soft tissue expansion. Tissue expansion was first described by Radovan [21, 22] as a method of creating soft tissue with similar color, texture, thickness, and sensation as the adjacent tissue with minimal scarring and little donor site morbidity. Neumann was the first who mentioned the potential to use tissue expansion for reconstructive surgery [22, 23]. Nowadays tissue expansion is a well-known technique for head and neck reconstructive surgery [24–27]. Soft tissue expansion is a physiological process that leads to the formation of new cells and growth of tissue [28] and allows us to gain extra soft tissue with similar color, texture and function to that of the adjacent tissues for covering grafts [29].

After the tissue expander is inserted, during the expansion process the tissue is under a persistent tensile stress; traction of the surrounding soft tissue leads to extra soft tissue volume [30–32]. Sub-periosteal implantation of the expander is usually preferred over extra-periosteal implantation because of its optimum soft tissue increase [33]. However, sub-periosteal implantation of the expander limits the nutritional supply to the bone [34].

Traditional tissue expanders are silicone envelopes with self-sealing injection ports. They are filled by serial saline injections through the ports at weekly intervals. Volume expansion of the expander puts tension on the overlying tissue [35]. These traditional tissue expanders are now known to be associated with complications because of their intermittent sudden expansion [36]; this lead to the development of osmotic tissue expanders (OTEs). The OTE was first described by Austad and Rose [37]. It was made of a semi-permeable membrane filled with hypertonic saline which leads to the entrance of the water by osmotic forces from the surrounding tissues into the expander. Wiese developed an osmotic self-inflating expander [38], which has been used successfully to expand the orbit in the management of enophthalmos, microphthalmos, and cryptophthalmos [39–41].

The osmotic self-filling expander is made of polymeric methyl methacrylate–vinylpyrrolidone which gains volume by absorbing body fluids [42, 43]. The purpose of this chapter is to present some examples of the application of this expander before bone graft augmentation.

2. Technique

We used OTE in various patients. In our study, we used OSMED (Ilmenau, Germany) self-inflating tissue expanders (**Figure 1**) prior to bone augmentation and evaluated its complications and problems.

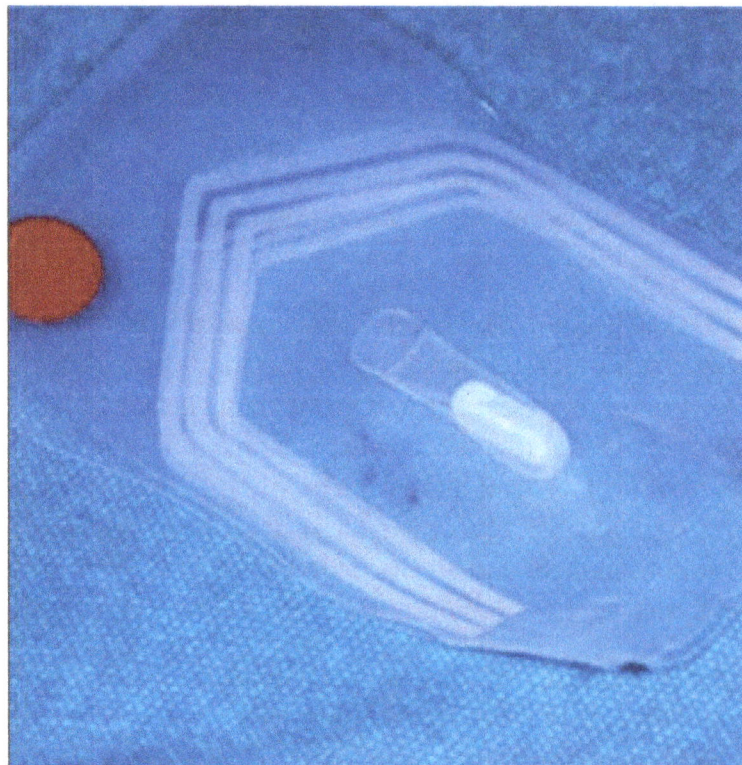

Figure 1. Osmed tissue expander.

2.1. Surgical technique

After making a full thickness incision, a sub-periosteal tunnel was prepared (**Figure 2**). After completion of the tunnel preparation, the tissue expander was placed under the tunnel flap while keeping the surgical field as dry as possible to reduce the risk of contamination with oral fluids. Wound closure was performed to minimize the leakage and contamination. The sutures were removed after 2 weeks. The tissue expanders were removed approximately 6–10 weeks later in the course of augmentation surgery; 1 g of intravenous cefazolin antibiotic was administered pre-operatively and continued every 6 h post-operatively for 24 h then it was replaced by 500 mg of oral cephalexin antibiotic taken every 6 h for the next 7 days. Chlorhexidine mouth-wash was used every 8 h post-operatively and was continued for 14 days.

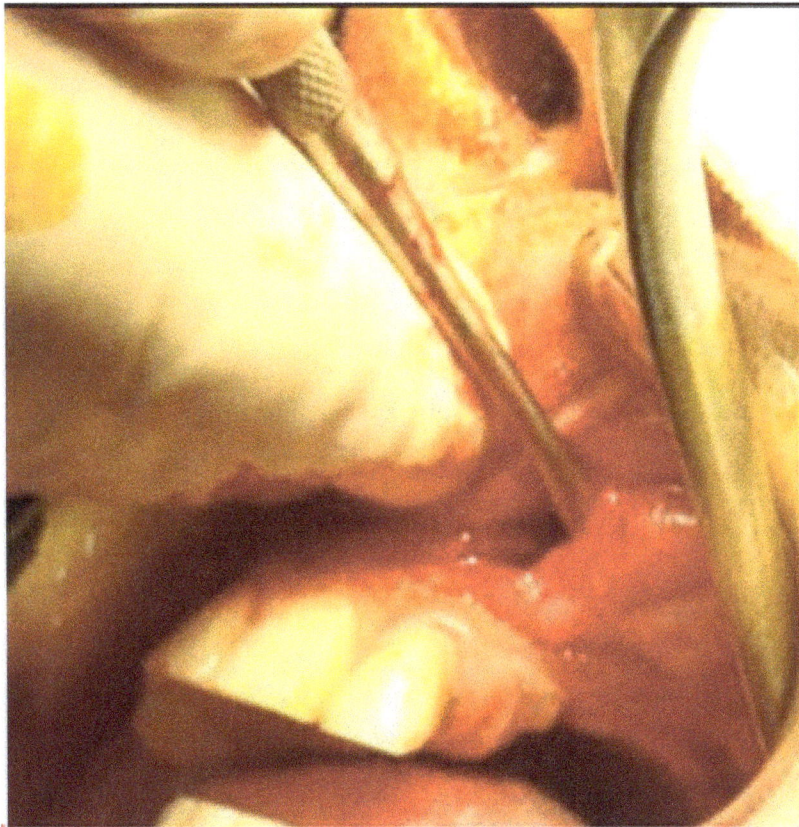

Figure 2. Subperiostal tunnel preparation.

3. Cases

3.1. Patient 1

A 23-year-old male had partial maxillectomy surgery on the left side due to central giant cell granuloma 12 years ago (**Figure 3**).

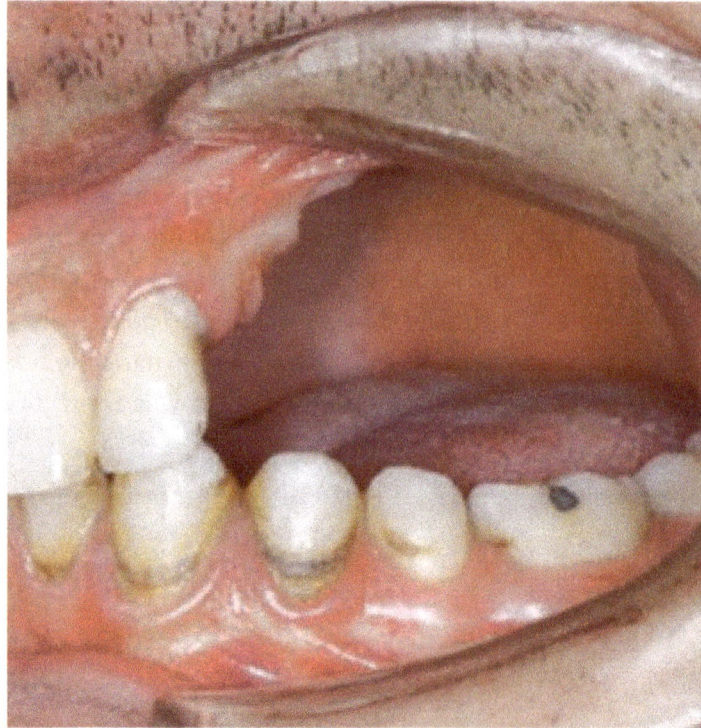

Figure 3. Partial maxillectomy of the left side.

In the first operation, an OSMED tissue expander cylinder 2.1 ml, with initial volume of 0.42 ml and final volume of 2.1 ml was placed sub-periosteally in the defect (**Figure 4**).

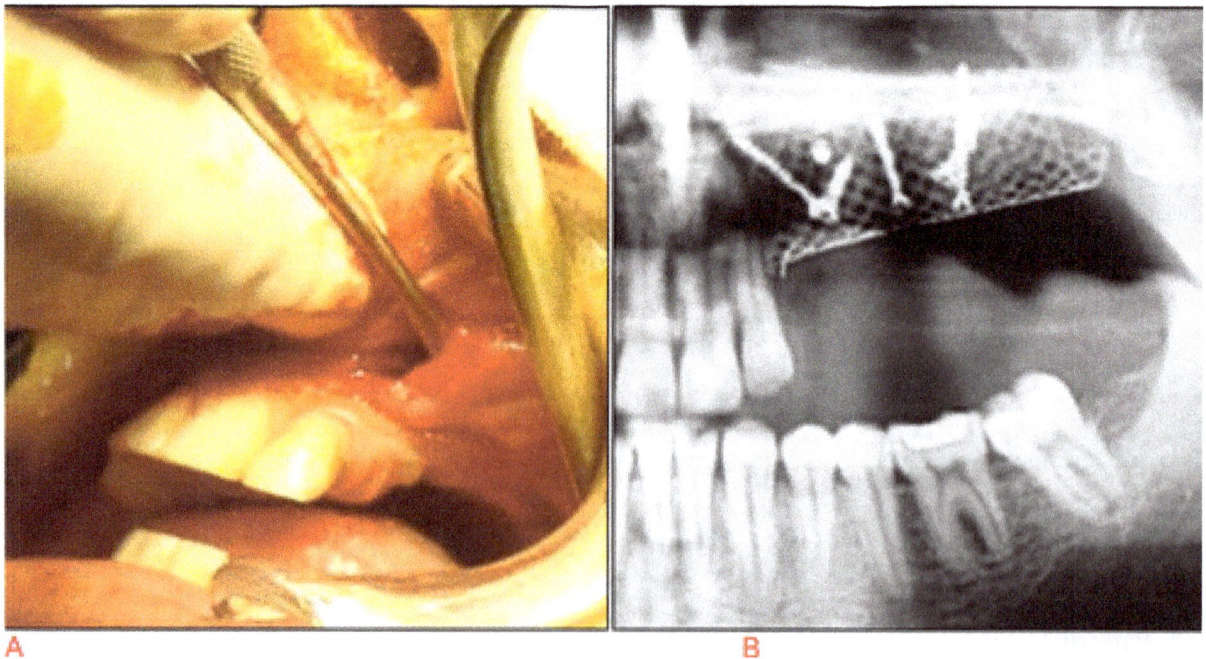

Figure 4. (A) OSMED tissue expander was placed sub-periosteally. (B) 10 weeks later, the tissue expander was removed and the bone was augmented.

In the second operation, done 10 weeks later, the tissue expander was removed and the bone was augmented by iliac bone graft (**Figure 5**).

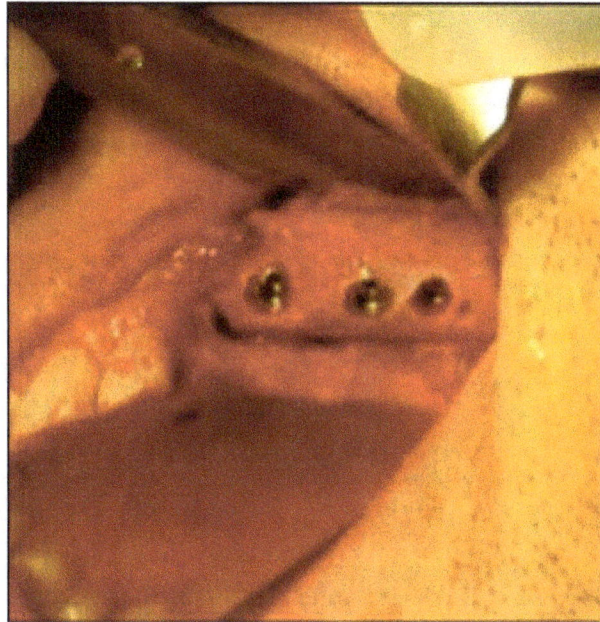

Figure 5. The tissue expander was removed and the bone augmented by iliac bone graft.

In the third operation, done 5 months later, the titanium mesh and fixation screws were removed and three dental implants were inserted (**Figure 6**). No post-operative complications were observed.

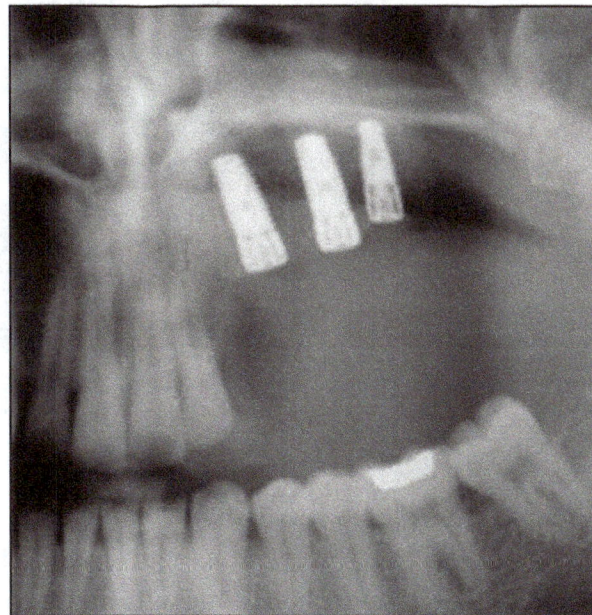

Figure 6. The titanium mesh and fixation screws removed and three dental implants were inserted.

3.2. Patient 2

A 54-year-old woman had severe mandibular atrophy. She had been edentulous for 30 years and had bone augmentation with iliac bone graft on the right side of the mandible 20 years ago. In the first operation, because of the lack of enough soft tissue and the presence of scar tissues from previous surgery, we used an OSMED tissue expander cylinder 1.3 ml, with initial volume of 0.25 ml and final volume of 1.3 ml (**Figure 7**).

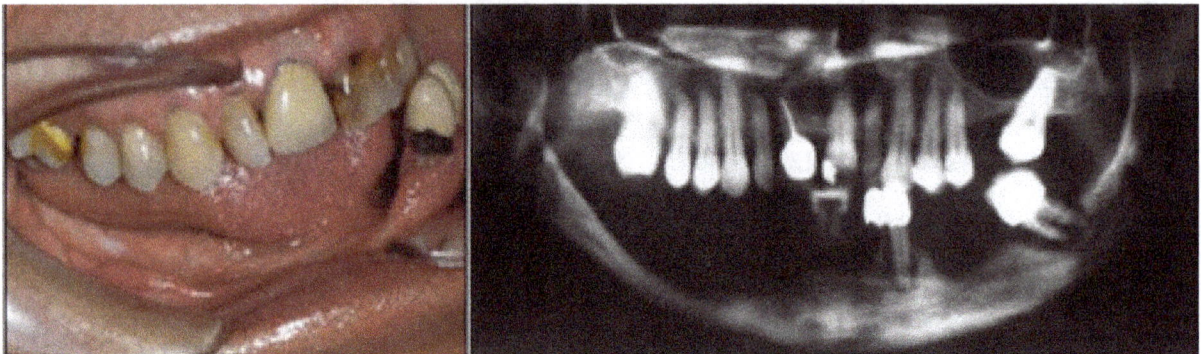

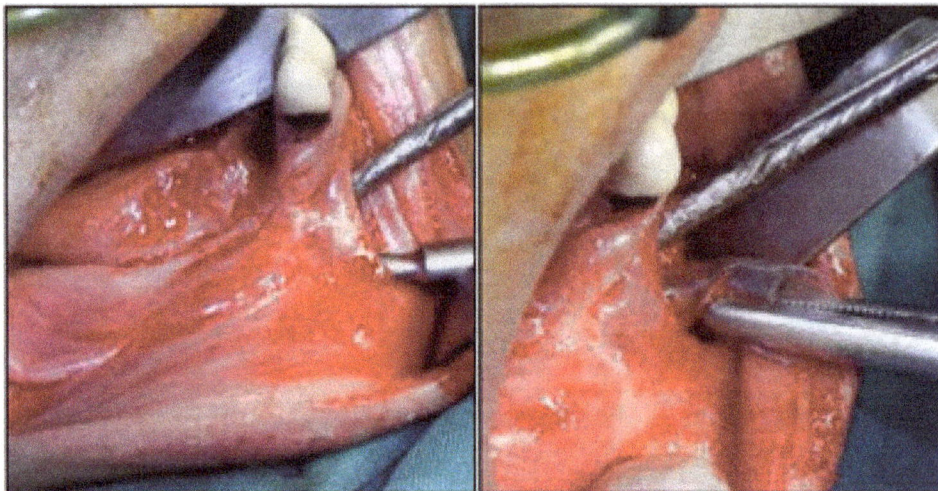

Figure 7. Severe mandibular atrophy. OSMED tissue expander cylinder placed in a sub-periosteal tunnel.

In the second operation, done 6 weeks later, the tissue expander was removed and the bone was augmented with iliac bone graft (**Figure 8**) and later dental implants were inserted (**Figure 9**). In this case, despite of the lack of enough soft tissue and the presence of scar tissues, the hard tissue was augmented vertically and desirable outcome and adequate bone volume for implant placement was achieved.

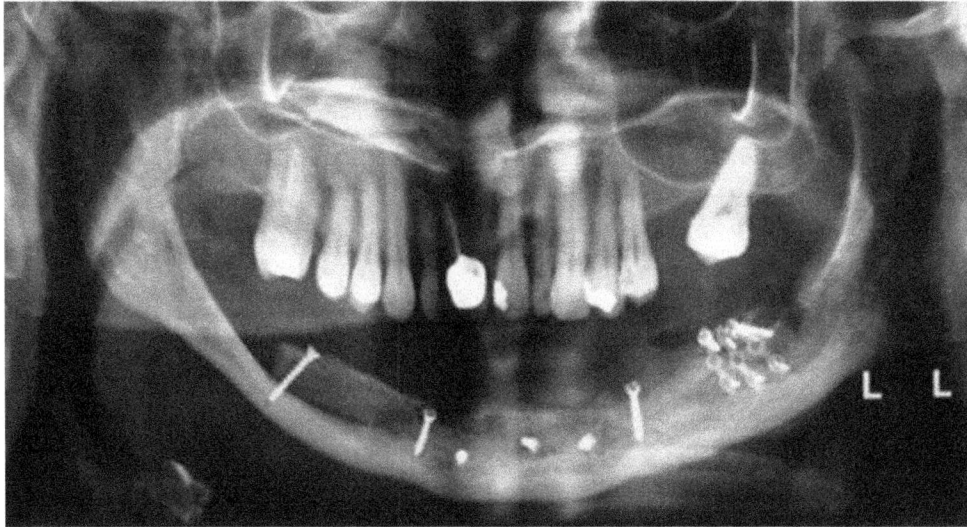

Figure 8. The bone was augmented with iliac bone graft.

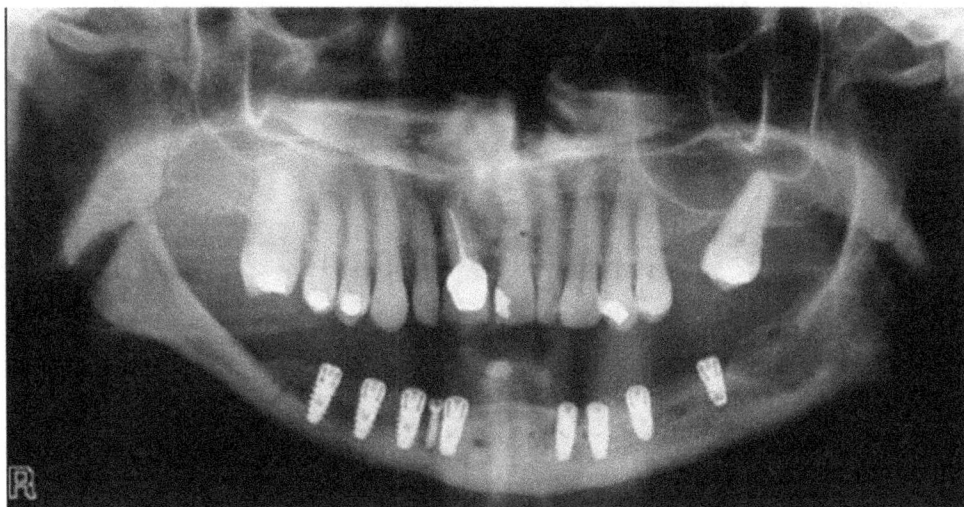

Figure 9. Later dental implants were inserted.

3.3. Patient 3

A 41-year-old woman had previous partial mandibular resection surgery due to an amelo-blastoma (**Figure 10**).

In the first operation, an OSMED tissue expander cylinder 2.1 ml was used. In the second operation, done 8 weeks later, the tissue expander was removed and the bone was augmented by iliac bone graft prior to dental implant insertion (**Figure 11**). In this case, due to the tension free closure of the soft tissue overlying the bone graft, postoperative complications were reduced and good results obtained.

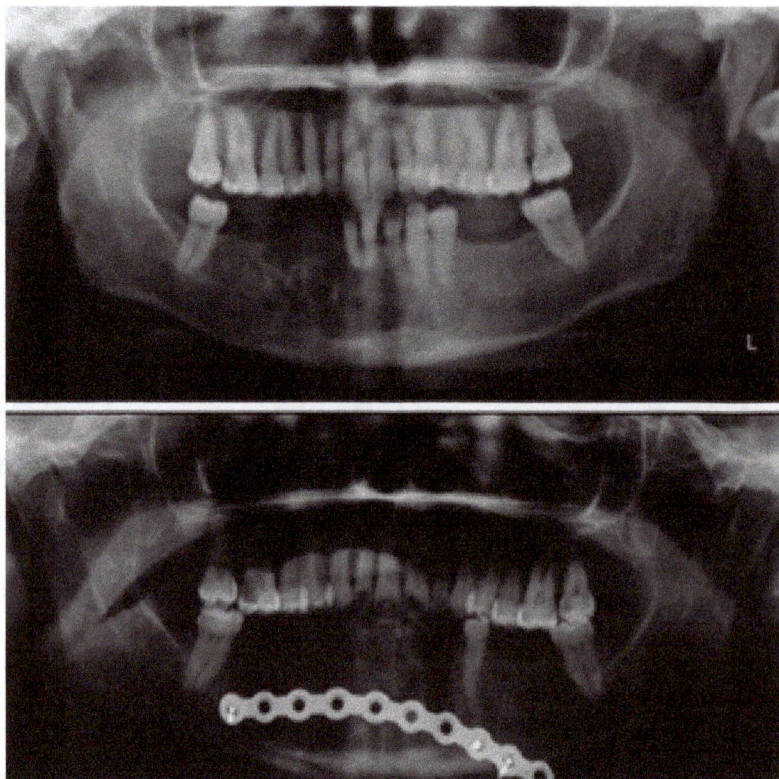

Figure 10. Ameloblastoma of the lower jaw. Resected.

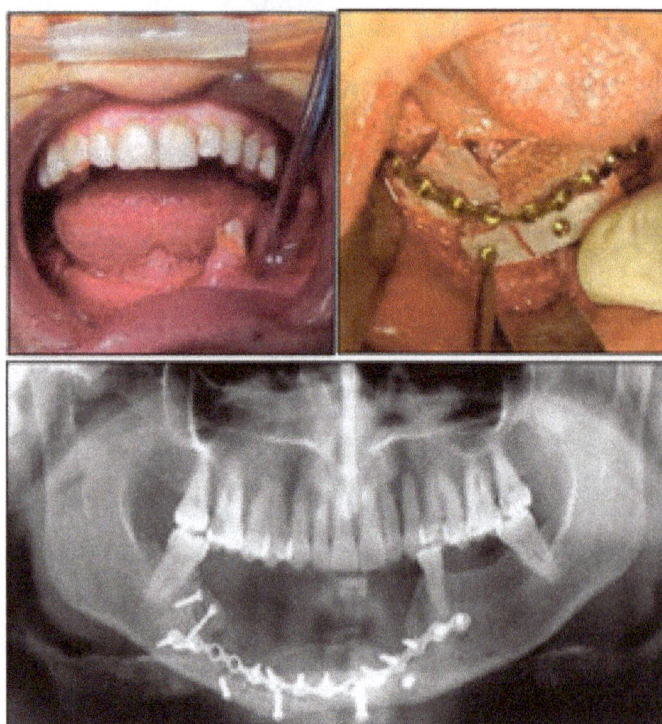

Figure 11. Left, Sub-periosteal tunnel preparation for tissue expander implantation Right, Bone augmentation was performed 8 weeks later Bottom, Panoramic view of the patient after bone augmentation.

4. Discussion

Soft tissue expansion has been used successfully for the reconstruction of soft tissue defects [44–47]. In case of inadequate normal soft tissue, new tissue should be created with the same color, texture and function as the adjacent tissue, which was first described by Neumann [48] for auricular reconstruction. In the head and neck area, tissue expansion has been used successfully for scalp, nose and ears [29, 30, 49, 50]. Intraoral soft tissue expanders have also been used prior to the bone augmentation in the case of inadequate soft tissue for primary tension free wound closure [51–56]. In their study they used classic forms of tissue expanders which were inflatable expanders inflated by weekly injections of saline. However, because of their sudden and intermittent volume increase, tissue hypoxia due to decreased blood flow to the area was reported [57]. Two types of expansion regimens are used clinically for classic tissue expansion namely 'conventional, prolonged expansion' for 1–3 months and 'intraoperative sustained limited expansion' [58, 59]. Some studies suggest that 'conventional, prolonged tissue expansion' can also be performed for 1–2 weeks without complications [60, 61]. The most common complications of soft tissue expansion are infection, dehiscence, hematoma, necrosis and failure [46, 47, 62–64]. When infection occurs, the expanders are usually removed to control the infection. Although several methods have been reported to salvage tissue expanders [65–67], usually substitution of the infected tissue expander with a new one is required.

By making a small incision as far as possible from the intended site for tissue expander insertion, the risk of dehiscence and failure is minimized [22, 29, 45]. Generally, in the same conditions, the smaller tissue expander is preferred over the larger one. Larger tissue expander usually require larger incisions with wider dissection and more undermining, which may increase the risk of dehiscence and also may cause scar expansion instead of normal tissue expansion [68]. As mentioned earlier, the expansion rate is important. Use of self-inflatable osmotic expander, has a gradual rate of expansion [43]. The early osmotic implants were made of a semi-permeable envelopes containing hypertonic liquid. Their expansion rates were rapid and were completed within the first 24–48 h following insertion and they were associated with more complications such as tissue ischemia and failure. Subsequent tissue expanders were made of dehydrated hydrogel in a silicone envelope with a more gradual expansion rate and lower complications [43, 69]. The OSMED self-inflating tissue expanders are made of a specially developed hydrogel that use the osmotic principle to gain volume. The hydrogel is made of co-polymers based on methyl methacrylate and N-vinyl pyrrolidone. Pre-operatively they are in their pre-expanded state and therefore are small, hard and easy to handle. After implantation, they start to absorb body fluid and grow consistently to a predefined shape and size. Their final volume depends on the product type and is between 3 and 12 fold their initial volume. The increase volume of the implant leads to an increase of soft tissue. Their expansion speed also differs by the product type. In some the tissue expander is delivered in a silicone shell, with an exact number and size of holes to assure gradual and consistent swelling of the device.

In this study, we used OSMED self-inflating tissue expander cylinder which is delivered in a silicone shell. The tissue expanders were placed sub-periosteally. It is reported that sub-periosteal implantation causes significant resorption of the underlying bone by impairing the micro-circulation of the underlying bone [33, 70–72], which was not observed in our patients. Periosteal-releasing incisions may reduce the blood supply to soft tissue flaps and increase the risk of dehiscence. The periosteal expansion facilitates a tension-free wound closure without the need to use any periosteal-releasing incisions [16]. Another strategy for minimizing the risk of intraoral dehiscence and infection [29] is keeping the incision small and away from the tissue expander, which may explain the low incidence of complications in our study and other reports [43]. It has been reported that slow and continuous expansion results in safe and effective generation of soft tissue and decreased incidence of intraoral dehiscence [38, 73]. In our study, the rate of expansion was slow enough not to cause any perforation of the soft tissue [74]. After expansion, the quality and quantity of expanded soft tissue was good enough to permit easy primary tension-free wound closure after major bone augmentation. The slow expansion will lead to slow and proper formation of new tissues over the time period [73].

5. Conclusion

In conclusion, our cases demonstrate that the use of tissue expander prior to bone augmentation can reduce the complications associated with non-OTE and lead to more predictable results.

Author details

Farzin Sarkarat[1], Farshid Kavandi[2*], Rouzbeh Kahali[1] and Mohammad Hosein Kalantar Motamedi[3]

*Address all correspondence to: farshid_kavandi@yahoo.com

1 Department of Oral and Maxillofacial Surgery, CMF Research Center, Buali Hospital, Islamic Azad University of Medical Sciences, Tehran, Iran

2 Department of Oral and Maxillofacial Surgery, Shahid Beheshti University of Medical Sciences, Tehran, Iran

3 Trauma Research Center, Baqiyatallah University of Medical Science and Islamic Azad University of Medical Sciences, Tehran, Iran

References

[1] Sebastian P, Thomas S, Varghese BT, Lype EM, Balagopal PG, Mathew PC. The submental island flap for reconstruction of intraoral defects in oral cancer patients. Oral Oncol 2008;44(11):1014–1018. Epub 2008 Jul 11.

[2] Wang HL, Boyapati L. "PASS" principles for predictable bone regeneration. Implant Dent 2006;15:8–17.

[3] Futran ND, Alsarraf R. Microvascular free-flap reconstruction in the head and neck. J Am Med Assoc 2000;284:1761–1763.

[4] Eckardt A, Meyer A, Laas U, Hausamen JE. Free flap reconstruction of head and neck defects—a clinical review of twenty years. Br J Oral Maxillofac Surg 2007;45:11–15.

[5] Urban IA, Jovanovic SA, Lozada JL. Vertical ridge augmentation using guided bone regeneration (GBR) in three clinical scenarios prior to implant placement: a retrospective study of 35 patients 12 to 72 months after loading. Int J Oral Maxillofac Implants 2009;24:502–510.

[6] Felice P, Marchetti C, Iezzi G, Piattelli A, Worthington H, Pellegrino G, Esposito M. Vertical ridge augmentation of the atrophic posterior mandible with interpositional bloc grafts: bone from the iliac crest vs. bovine anorganic bone. Clinical and histological results up to one year after loading from a randomized-controlled clinical trial. Clin Oral Implants Res 2009;20:1386–1393.

[7] Canullo L, Malagnino VA. Vertical ridge augmentation around implants by e-PTFE titanium reinforced membrane and bovine bone matrix: a 24- to 54-month study of 10 consecutive cases. Int J Oral Maxillofac Implants 2008;23:858–866.

[8] Merli M, Migani M, Esposito M. Vertical ridge augmentation with autogenous bone grafts: resorbable barriers supported by ostheosynthesis plates versus titanium reinforced barriers. A preliminary report of a blinded, randomized controlled clinical trial. Int J Oral Maxillofac Implants 2007;22:373–382.

[9] Barone A, Covani U. Maxillary alveolar ridge reconstruction with nonvascularized autogenous block bone: clinical results. J Oral Maxillofac Surg 2007;65:2039–2046.

[10] Cordaro L, Amade DS, Cordaro M. Clinical results of alveolar ridge augmentation with mandibular block bone grafts in partially edentulous patients prior to implant placement. Clin Oral Implants Res 2002;13:103–11.

[11] Lundgren S, Sjostrom M, Nystrom E, Sennerby L. Strategies in reconstruction of the atrophic maxilla with autogenous bone grafts and endosseous implants. Periodontology 2000 2008;47:143–161.

[12] von Arx T, Kurt B. Implant placement and simultaneous ridge augmentation using autogenous bone and a micro titanium mesh: a prospective clinical study with 20 implants. Clin Oral Implants Res 1999;10:24–33.

[13] Esposito M, Grusovin MG, Maghaireh H, Coulthard P, Worthington HV. Interventions for replacing missing teeth: management of soft tissues for dental implants. Cochrane Database Syst Rev 2007:CD006697.

[14] Jivraj S, Chee W. Treatment planning of implants in the esthetics zone. Br Dent J 2006;201:77–89.

[15] Rothamel D, Schwarz F, Herten M, Ferrari D, Mischkowski RA, Sager M, Becker J. Vertical ridge augmentation using xenogenous bone blocks: a histomorphometric study in dogs. Int J Oral Maxillofac Implants 2009;24:243–250.

[16] Abrahamsson P, Isaksson S, Gordh M, Andersson G. Onlay bone grafting of the mandible after periosteal expansion with an osmotic tissue expander: an experimental study in rabbits. Clin Oral Implants Res 2010;21(12):1404–10.

[17] Nakayama Y, Soeda S, Kasai Y. The importance of arterial inflow in the distal side of a flap: an experimental investigation. Plast Reconstr Surg 1982;69:61–67.

[18] McLean TN, Smith BA, Morrison EC, Nasjleti CE, Caffesse RG. Vascular changes following mucoperiosteal flap surgery: a fluorescein angiography study in dogs. J Periodontol 1995;66:205–210.

[19] Morris SF, Pang CY, Zhong A, Boyd B. Forrest CR. Assessment of ischemia-induced reperfusion injury in the pig latissimus dorsi myocutaneous flap model. Plast Reconstr Surg 1993;92:1162–1172.

[20] Carroll WR, Esclamado RM. Ischemia/reperfusion injury in microvascular surgery. Head Neck 2000;22:700–713.

[21] Radovan C. Breast reconstruction after mastectomy using the temporary expander. Plast Reconstr Surg 1982;69:195–208.

[22] Radovan C. Tissue expansion in soft-tissue reconstruction. Plast Reconstr Surg 1984;74:482–92.

[23] Iconomou TG, Michelow BJ, Zuker RM. Tissue expansion in the pediatric patient. Ann Plast Surg 1993;31:134–40.

[24] Menard RM, Moore MH, David DJ. Tissue expansion in the reconstruction of Tessier craniofacial clefts: a series of 17 patients. Plast Reconstr Surg 1999;103(3):779–86.

[25] Zaal LH, van der Horst CM. Results of the early use of tissue expansion for giant congenital melanocytic naevi on the scalp and face. J Plast Reconstr Aesthet Surg 2009;62(2):216–20.

[26] Mahoney EJ, Dolan RW, Choi EE, et al. Surgical reconstruction of lentigomaligna defects. Arch Facial Plast Surg 2005;7(5):342–6.

[27] Hurvitz KA, Rosen H, Meara JG. Pediatric cervicofacial tissue expansion. Int J Pediatr Otorhinolaryngol 2005;69(11):1509–13.

[28] van Rappard JH, Molenaar J, van Doorn K, Sonneveld GJ, Borghouts JM. Surface-area increase in tissue expansion. Plast Reconstr Surg 1988;82:833–9.

[29] Wieslander JB. Tissue expansion in the head and neck. A 6-year review. Scand J Plast Reconstr Surg Hand Surg 1991;25:47–56.

[30] Antonyshyn O, Gruss JS, Zuker R, Mackinnon SE. Tissue expansion in head and neck reconstruction. Plast Reconstr Surg 1988;82:58–68.

[31] Bennett RG, Hirt M. A history of tissue expansion. Concepts, controversies, and complications. J Dermatol Surg Oncol 1993;19:1066–1073.

[32] Bascom DA, Wax KA. Tissue expansion in the head and neck: current state of the art. Curr Opin Otolaryngol Head Neck Surg 2002;10:273–277.

[33] Rucker M, Binger T, Deltcheva K, Menger MD. Reduction of midfacial periosteal perfusion failure by subperiosteal versus supraperiosteal dissection. J Oral Maxillofac Surg 2005;63:87–92.

[34] Chanavaz M. Anatomy and histophysiology of the periosteum: quantification of the periosteal blood supply to the adjacent bone with 85Sr and gamma spectrometry. J Oral Implantol 1995;21:214–219.

[35] Argenta LC. Tissue expansion. In: Aston SJ, Beasley RW, editors. Thorne CHM Plastic Surgery. 5th edn. New York: Lippincott-Raven; 1997. p. 91.

[36] Cunha MS, Nakamoto HA, Herson MR, et al. Tissue expander complications in plastic surgery. A 10-year experience. Rev Hosp Clin Fac Med Sao Paulo 2002;57:93–97.

[37] Austad ED, Rose GL. A self-inflating tissue expander. Plast Reconstr Surg 1982;70:588–94.

[38] Wiese KG. Osmotically induced tissue expansion with hydrogels: a new dimension in tissue expansion? A preliminary report. J Craniomaxillofac Surg 1993;21:309–13.

[39] Downes R, Lavin M, Collin R. Hydrophyllic expanders for the congenital anophthalmic socket. Adv Ophthalmic Plast Reconstr Surg 1992;9:57–61.

[40] Wiese KG, Vogel M, Guthoff R, et al. Treatment of congenital anophthalmos with self-inflating polymer expanders: a new method. J Craniomaxillofac Surg 1999;27:72–6.

[41] Gundlach KK, Guthoff RF, Hingst VH, et al. Expansion of the socket and orbit for congenital clinical anophthalmia. Plast Reconstr Surg 2005;116:1214–22.

[42] Berge SJ, Wiese KG, von Lindern JJ, Niederhagen B, Appel T, Reich RH. Tissue expansion using osmotically active hydrogel systems for direct closure of the donor defect of the radial forearm flap. Plast Reconstr Surg 2001;108:1–5 (discussion 6–7).

[43] Ronert MA, Hofheinz H, Manassa E, Asgarouladi H, Olbrisch RR. The beginning of a new era in tissue expansion: self-filling osmotic tissue expander—four-year clinical experience. Plast Reconstr Surg 2004;114:1025–1031.

[44] Cullen KW, Powell B. Tissue expanders in surgery. Br J Clin Pract 1989;43:75–77.

[45] Houpt P, Dijkstra R. Tissue expansion in reconstructive surgery. Neth J Surg 1988;40:13–16.

[46] Manders EK, Schenden MJ, Furrey JA, Hetzler PT, Davis TS, Graham WP, III. Soft-tissue expansion: concepts and complications. Plast Reconstr Surg 1984;74:493–507.

[47] Neale HW, Kurtzman LC, Goh KB, Billmire DA, Yakuboff KP, Warden G. Tissue expanders in the lower face and anterior neck in pediatric burn patients: limitations and pitfalls. Plast Reconstr Surg 1993;91:624–631.

[48] Neumann CG. The expansion of an area of skin by progressive distention of a subcutaneous balloon; use of the method for securing skin for subtotal reconstruction of the ear. Plast Reconstr Surg 1957;19:124–130.

[49] Argenta LC. Controlled tissue expansion in reconstructive surgery. Br J Plast Surg 1984;37:520–529.

[50] Argenta LC, VanderKolk CA. Tissue expansion in craniofacial surgery. Clin Plast Surg 1987;14:143–153.

[51] Zeiter DJ, Ries WL, Weir TL, Mishkin DJ, Sanders JJ. The use of a soft tissue expander in an alveolar bone ridge augmentation for implant placement. Int J Periodontics Restor Dent 1998;18:403–409.

[52] Lew D, Amos EA, Unhold GP. An open procedure for placement of a tissue expander over the atrophic alveolar ridge. J Oral Maxillofac Surg 1988;46:161–166.

[53] Lew D, Hinkle RM, Collins SF. Use of subperiosteal implants with distal filling ports in the correction of the atrophic alveolar ridge. Int J Oral Maxillofac Surg 1991;20:15–17.

[54] Bahat O, Handelsman M. Controlled tissue expansion in reconstructive periodontal surgery. Int J Periodontics Restor Dent 1991;11:32–47.

[55] Lew D, Amos EL, Shroyer JV, III. The use of a subperiosteal tissue expander in rib reconstruction of an atrophic mandible. J Oral Maxillofac Surg 1988;46:229–232.

[56] Wittkampf AR. Short-term experience with the subperiosteal tissue expander in reconstruction of the mandibular alveolar ridge. J Oral Maxillofac Surg 1989;47:469–474.

[57] Pietila JP. Tissue expansion and skin circulation. Simultaneous monitoring by laser Doppler flowmetry and transcutaneous oximetry. Scand J Plast Reconstr Surg Hand Surg 1990;24:135–140.

[58] Machida BK, Liu-Shindo M, Sasaki GH, Rice DH, Chandrasoma P. Immediate versus chronic tissue expansion. Ann Plast Surg 1991;26:227–231.

[59] Saski GH. Intra operative sustained limited expansion (ISLE) as an immediate recon-structive technique. Clin Plast Surg 1987;14:563–573.

[60] Mustoe TA, Bartell TH, Garner WL. Physical, biomechanical, histologic, and biochem-ical effects of rapid versus conventional tissue expansion. Plast Reconstr Surg 1989;83:687–691.

[61] Timmenga EJ, Schoorl R, Klopper PJ. Biomechanical and histomorphological changes in expanded rabbit skin. Br J Plast Surg 1990;43:101–106.

[62] Cunha MS, Nakamoto HA, Herson MR, Faes JC, Gemperli R, Ferreira MC. Tissue expander complications in plastic surgery: a 10-year experience. Rev Hosp Clin Fac Med Sao Paulo 2002;57:93–97.

[63] Bozkurt A, Groger A, O'Dey D, et al. Retrospective analysis of tissue expansion in reconstructive burn surgery: evaluation of complication rates. Burns 2008;34(8):1113–1118.

[64] Tavares Filho JM, Belerique M, Franco D, Porchat CA, Franco T. Tissue expansion in burn sequelae repair. Burns 2007;33(2):246–251.

[65] Yii NW, Khoo CTK. Salvage of infected expander prostheses in breast reconstruction. Plast Reconstr Surg 2003;111:1087–1092.

[66] Chun JK, Schulman MR. The infected breast prosthesis after mastectomy reconstruc-tion: successful salvage of nine implants in eight consecutive patients. Plast Reconstr Surg 2007;120:581–589.

[67] Kendrick AS, Chase CW. Salvage of an infected breast tissue expander with an implant sizer and negative pressure wound management. Plast Reconstr Surg 2008;121:138e–139e.

[68] Hallock GG. Safety of clinical overinflation of tissue expanders. Plast Reconstr Surg 1995;96:153–157.

[69] Anwander T, Schneider M, Gloger W, et al. Investigation of the expansion properties of osmotic expanders with and without silicone shells in animals. Plast Reconstr Surg 2007;120:590–595.

[70] Stuehmer C, Rucker M, Schumann P, Bormann KH, Harder Y, Sinikovic B, Gellrich NC. Osseous alterations at the interface of hydrogel expanders and underlying bone. J Craniomaxillofac Surg 2009;37:258–262.

[71] Schaser KD, Zhang L, Haas NP, Mittlmeier T, Duda G, Bail HJ. Temporal profile of microvascular disturbances in rat tibialperiosteum following closed soft tissue trauma. Langenbeck's Arch Surg 2003;388:323–330.

[72] Hemmer KM, Marsh JL, Picker S. Calvarial erosion after scalp expansion. Ann Plast Surg 1987;19:454–459.

[73] Wiese KG, Heinemann DE, Ostermeier D, Peters JH. Biomaterial properties and biocompatibility in cell culture of a novel self inflating hydrogel tissue expander. J Biomed Mater Res 2001;54:179–188.

[74] Kaner D, Friedmann A. Soft tissue expansion with self-filling osmotic tissue expanders before vertical ridge augmentation: a proof of principle study. J Clin Periodontol 2010.

5

Three-Dimensional Printing: A Novel Technology for Use in Oral and Maxillofacial Operations

Seied Omid Keyhan, Sina Ghanean,
Alireza Navabazam, Arash Khojasteh and
Mohammad Hosein Amirzade Iranaq

Abstract

Three-dimensional (3D) printing is cited as "a novel, fascinating, future builder technology" in many papers and articles. Use of this technology in the field of medicine and especially oral and maxillofacial surgery is expanding. The type of manufacturing systems, materials, cost-effectiveness, and also bio-printing, with studies from around the world today, make this field a "hot-topic" in reconstructive and regenerative surgery. This chapter evaluates the latest updates and scientific uses of 3D printing.

Keywords: Rapid prototyping, three-dimensional printing, reconstructive surgery, oral, maxillofacial surgery

1. Introduction

Three-dimensional printing (3D), also known as rapid prototyping (RP), was first introduced in the 1980s. During the past three decades, enormous changes and developments have been made by scientists modifying this technology, materials, and accuracy. Within the field of craniofacial surgery, 3D surgical models have been used as templates to harvest bone grafts, tailoring bioprosthetic implants, plate bending, cutting guides for osteotomies, and intraoperative oral splints. Using 3D models and guides has been shown to shorten the operative time and reduce the complications associated with it. The ultimate goal of any surgical procedure is to improve peri-operative form and function and to minimize operative and postoperative morbidity. Many exciting and new technological advances have opened a new era in the field of oral and maxillofacial surgery over the last years, and 3D printing is among the most novel. The aim of this chapter is to introduce 3D printing method and its role in contemporary oral and maxillofacial surgery and to review different applications and benefits of 3D printing-assisted surgeries in the oral and maxillofacial region.

2. History and benefits

Three-dimensional printing has been utilized in diverse aspects of manufacturing to produce different objects from guns, boats, and food to models of unborn babies. From over 1450 articles related to 3D printing listed in PubMed, nearly a third of them were published in the last 2 years [1].

3D printing is a manufacturing process wherein objects are fabricated in a layering method during fusing or depositing different materials such as plastic, metal, ceramics, powders, liquids, or even living cells to build a 3D structure [2, 3]. It is a process of generating physical models from digital layouts [4, 5]. This technology demonstrates a technique where a product designed via a computer-aided scheme is manufactured in a layer-by-layer system [6]. This process is also known as RP, solid freeform technology (SFF), or additive manufacturing (AM) [7].

3D printing techniques are not new and have existed since 30 years ago [8–10]. This technology was first introduced and invented by Charles Hull in 1986, and at first it was utilized in the engineering and automobile industry for manufacturing polyurethane frameworks for different models, pieces, and instruments [11]. Originally, Hull employed the phrase "Stereo-lithography" in his US Patent 4,575,330, termed "Apparatus for Production of Three – Dimensional Objects by Stereolithography" published in 1986. Stereolithography (SL) technique included subjoining layers over the top of each other, by curing photopolymers with UV lasers [12, 13].

Since then, 3D models have been used for a diversity of different objectives. Since 1986, this process has started to accelerate and has honored recognition globally and has influenced different arenas, such as medicine. The developing agora for 3D desktop printers encourages wide-ranging experimentations in all fields. Generally, medical indications of these printers are treatment planning, prosthesis implant fabrications, medical training, and other usages [4]. Having being used in the military, food industry, and arts, RP has received much attention in the field of surgery in the last 10 years [6, 14]. The pioneering usage of SL in oral and maxillofacial surgery was by Brix and Lambrecht in 1985. Later, this technique was used by them for treatment planning in craniofacial surgery [15]. In 1990, SL was used by Mankovich et al. for treating patients having craniofacial deformities [16, 17]. They used it to simulate bony anatomy of the cranium using computed tomography (CT) with complete internal components [17, 18].

By aiding in complex craniofacial reconstructions, 3D printing has recently earned reputation in medicine and surgical fields [19–21]. Today, maxillofacial surgery can benefit from additive manufacturing in various aspects and different clinical cases [22]. This technique can help with bending plates, manufacturing templates for bone grafts, tailoring implants, osteotomy guides, and intraoperative occlusal splints [23–27]. RP can shorten surgery duration and simplify pre- and intraoperative decisions. It has enhanced efficacy and preciseness of surgeries (**Table 1**) [10].

Diagnosis and treatment planning
Direct visualization of anatomic structures
Surgical guides/templates
Surgical practice/rehearsal
Designing incisions
Surgical resections
Assessment of bony defects for grafting
Adaptation/pre-bending of reconstruction plates
Fabrication of custom prostheses
TMJ prostheses, distraction devices, fixation devices
Decreased surgical time, anesthesia time, wound exposure duration
More predictable results
Improved colleague communication
Educational tool for patients

Table 1. Uses of 3D models [22].

3. Manufacturing process and types of models

There are different technologies introduced for 3D printing. Binder jetting (BJ), electron beam melting (EBM), fused deposition modeling (FDM), indirect processes, laser melting (LM), laser sintering (LS), material jetting (MJ), photopolymer jetting (PJ), and SL are well-known technologies of 3D printing [14, 28, 29]. There are many different 3D printing techniques. Benefits and disadvantages are factors inherent to each technology system [14]. Among this variety of different techniques, there is a huge demand for oral and maxillofacial surgery for SL, FDM, and PJ [1, 28, 30]. **Table 2** summarizes some different three-dimensional printing technologies.

3.1. Stereolithography (SL)

The initial 3D printing technique SL began in the late 1980s [31]. The original SL uses a laser beam for resin polymerization in two-dimensional patterns [32]. Being the pioneering additive manufacturing method, SL produces 3D objects by curing layers of liquid photopolymer or epoxy resin with a low-power UV laser [13]. SL projects a UV laser to a cross section of a single layer of the resin onto a photopolymer resulting in the setting of the layer. This is repeated until fabricating all zones of the product [1]. This technique utilizes a mirror to guide the laser to the surface in a layer-by-layer manner. Furthermore, the 3D device projects it on the surface resins. This procedure is done from the base to the surface (**Figure 1**) [14, 33].

Techniques	Advantages	Disadvantages
Light cured resin		
1. Stereolithography (SL) —Light-sensitive polymer cured layer by layer by a scanning laser in a vat of liquid polymer	Rapid fabrication. Able to create complex shapes with high feature resolution. Lower cost materials if used in bulk	Only available with light curable liquid polymers. Support materials must be removed. Resin is messy and can cause skin sensitization and may be irritant by contact and inhalation. Limited shelf life and vat life. Cannot be heat sterilized. High-cost technology
2. Photojet—Light-sensitive polymer is jetted onto a build platform from an inkjet-type print head and cured layer by layer on an incrementally descending platform	Relatively fast. High-resolution, high-quality finish possible. Multiple materials are available with various colors and physical properties including elastic materials. Lower cost technology	Tenacious support material can be difficult to remove completely. Support material may cause skin irritation. Cannot be heat sterilized. High- cost materials
3. DLP (digital light processing)—Liquid resin is cured layer by layer by a projector light source. The object is built upside down on an incrementally elevating platform	Good accuracy, smooth surfaces, relatively fast. Lower cost technology	Light curable liquid polymers and wax-like materials for casting. Support materials must be removed. Resins are messy, can cause skin sensitization, and may be irritant by contact. Limited shelf life and vat life. Cannot be heat sterilized. Higher cost materials
Powder binder		
Plaster or cementaceous material set by drops of (colored) water from "inkjet" print head. Object built layer by layer in a powder bed, on an incrementally descending platform	Lower cost materials and technology. Can print in color. Unset material provides support. Relatively fast process. Safe materials	Low resolution. Messy powder. Low strength. Cannot be soaked or heat sterilized
Sintered powder		
Selective laser sintering (SLS) for polymers —Object built layer by layer in powder bed. Heated build chamber raises temperature of material to just below melting point. Scanning laser then sinters powder layer by layer in a descending bed	Range of polymeric materials including nylon, elastomers, and composites. Strong and accurate parts. Self-supported process. Polymeric materials—commonly nylon may be autoclaved. Printed object may	Significant infrastructure required, e.g., compressed air, climate control. Messy powders. Lower cost in bulk. Inhalation risk. High-cost technology. Rough surface

Techniques	Advantages	Disadvantages
	have full mechanical functionality. Lower cost materials if used in large volume	
Selective laser sintering (SLS) — for metals and metal alloys. Also described as selective laser melting (SLM) or direct metal laser sintering (DMLS). Scanning laser sinters metal powder layer by layer in a cold build chamber as the build platform descends. Support structure used to tether objects to build platform	High-strength objects can control porosity. Variety of materials including titanium, titanium alloys, cobalt chrome, stainless steel. Metal alloy may be recycled. Fine detail possible	Elaborate infrastructure requirements. Extremely costly technology. Moderately costly materials. Dust and nanoparticle condensate may be hazardous to health. Explosive risk. Rough surface. Elaborate post-processing is required: Heat treatment to relieve internal stresses in printed objects. Hard to remove support materials. Relatively slow process
Electron beam melting (EBM, Arcam). Heated build chamber. Powder sintered layer by layer by scanning electron beam on descending build platform	High-temperature process, so no support or heat treatment needed afterward. High speed. Dense parts with controlled porosity	Extremely costly technology moderately costly materials. Dust may be hazardous to health. Explosive risk. Rough surface. Less post -processing required. Lower resolution
Thermoplastic		
Fused deposition modeling (FDM) First 3DP technology, most used in "home" printers. Thermoplastic material extruded through nozzle onto build platform	High porosity. Variable mechanical strength. Low-to-mid-range cost materials and equipment . Low accuracy in low-cost equipment. Some materials may be heat sterilized	Low cost but limited materials— only thermoplastics. Limited shape complexity for biological materials. Support material must be removed

Table 2. 3D printing modalities and materials [14].

It is necessary to extract waste materials manually from the eventual outcome [34–36]. Nowadays, SL is known as the gold standard in 3D manufacturing with yield resolutions up to 0.025 mm. SL is reliable in reconstruction of internal frameworks and is more efficient in fabricating larger objects [37]. SL is largely accepted to have the best surfacing and the most accuracy of any 3D technology. Materials used in this system must be to some degree brittle and light [38, 39]. Acrylics and epoxies are commonly used for this method [40]. However, SL still requires manual handling after fabrication, and the process lasts more than a day to be completed. SL is more expensive than other techniques due to materials used, and the printer is considered more expensive due to the high cost of the raw materials and device maintenance [23, 41]. SL is largely utilized for producing implant drill guides [14]. The ability to build complex and detailed structures, extraction of waste resin without difficulty, and extremely high resolution (~1.2 um) are considered main advantages of SL [42] feature.

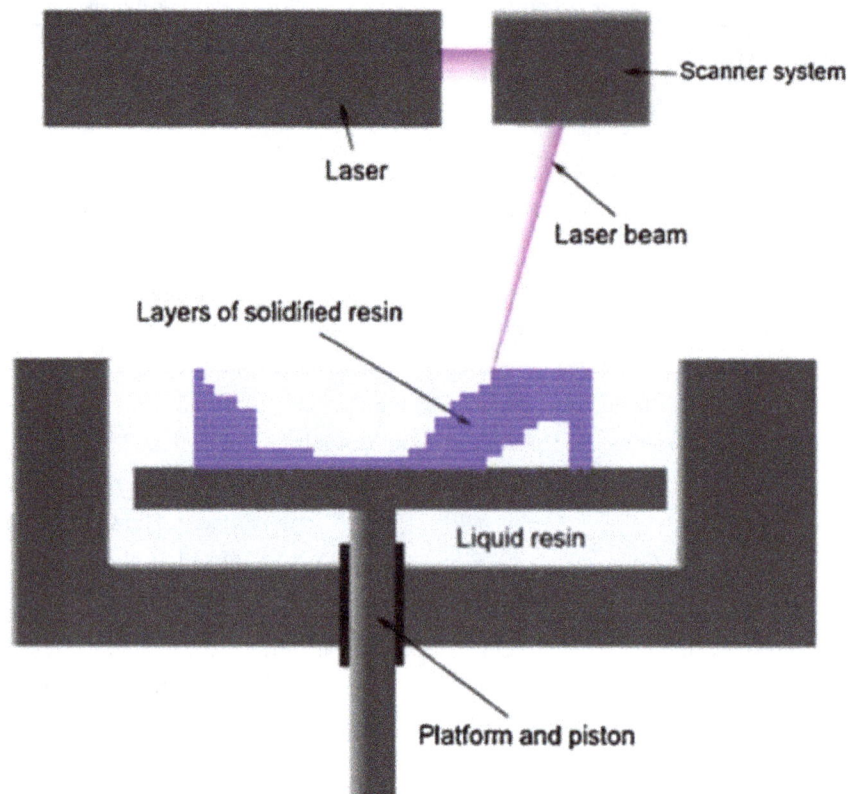

Figure 1. Schematic view of SL [115].

3.2. Fused deposition modeling

FDM uses a similar principle to SL in that it builds models on a layer-by-layer basis. When there is a discussion about cost-effectiveness, FDM is considered among the most utilized consumer 3D printing methods [16, 43, 44]. In FDM, a melted filament of thermoplastic material is extruded from a nozzle moving in the x-y plane and solidifies upon deposition on a build plate [45]. The build plate is lowered by 0.1 mm after each layer reappears. The process is repeated until the final product is produced. The most frequently used raw materials in FDM printers are acrylonitrile-butadiene-styrene (ABS) and polylactic acid (PLA) materials known for being key components of scaffold structures used for "bioprinting" [40].

Notable disadvantage and shortcoming for FDM is disability to form complex structures and most anatomical structures with complex shapes. For manufacturing a clean product, hollow internal structures or blind-ended openings are especially troublesome. Almost all household FDM printers are currently limited in mono-color and mono-material for manufacturing. However, this can be overcome by recently developed dual-extruder technology. In this technology, two filaments of different colors or materials can be extruded from a common printer head. MakerBot Replicator 2X Experimental (MakerBot Industries, New York, NY, USA), Cube 3 (3D Systems, Rock Hill, SC, USA), and Creatr x1 (Leapfrog, Emeryville, CA, USA) are known for this ability. Even more, the second extruder can be configured to build support structures using MakerBot Dissolvable Filament (MakerBot Industries), made of high-impact polystyrene (HIPS) [6, 46].

Support structures are required for FDM models such as SL as thermoplastic needs time to harden and also the layers to bond together [47]. Since multiple extrusion nozzles can be used in FDM, each with a different material, there is no theoretical restriction on compositional gradients in all three dimensions for FDM. High porosity due to the laydown pattern and good mechanical strength are notable and key advantages of FDM (**Figure 2**).

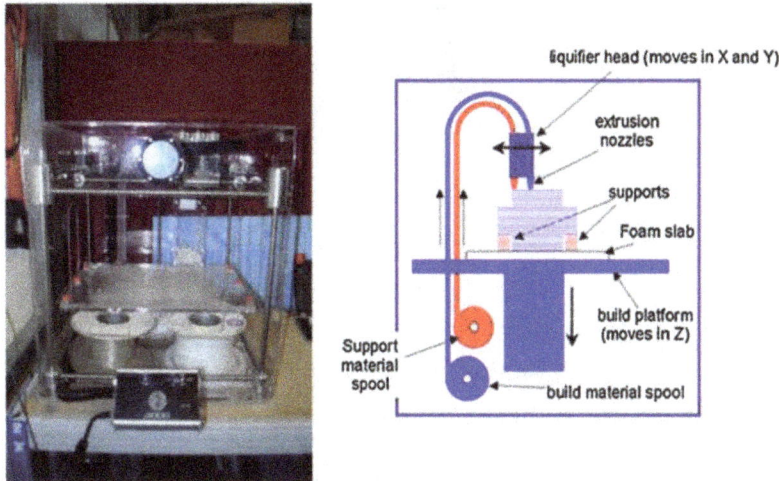

Figure 2. Schematic view of FDM [40].

3.3. PolyJet modeling

Multijet modeling printing, also known as MultiJet Printing (3D Systems, Rock Hill, SC, USA) or PolyJet Technology (Stratasys, Edina, MN, USA), is similar to SL; the difference is that the liquid photopolymer is immediately cured by UV light [48]. Multijet modeling printing can manufacture prototypes with high resolution (16 μ) that is comparable to or even better than SL. The advantage is the capacity to print in multiple materials for the desired degree of tensile strength and durability. An MJM printer is easier to maintain than an SL system. On the contrary, a disadvantage is the high price of these printers which makes MJM(Multi Jet Modeling) more suitable for large-scale productions rather than for office-based applications (**Figure 3**) [6].

The drawback is that the equipment and materials are costly to purchase and run, and the support materials can be tenacious and rather unpleasant to remove. They are useful for printing dental or anatomical study models, but these are expensive when produced. A particular advantage of this technology is that the use of multiple print heads allows simultaneous printing with different materials, and graduated mixtures of materials, makes it possible to vary the properties of the printed object, which may for example have flexible and rigid parts, for the production of indirect orthodontic bracket splints [14].

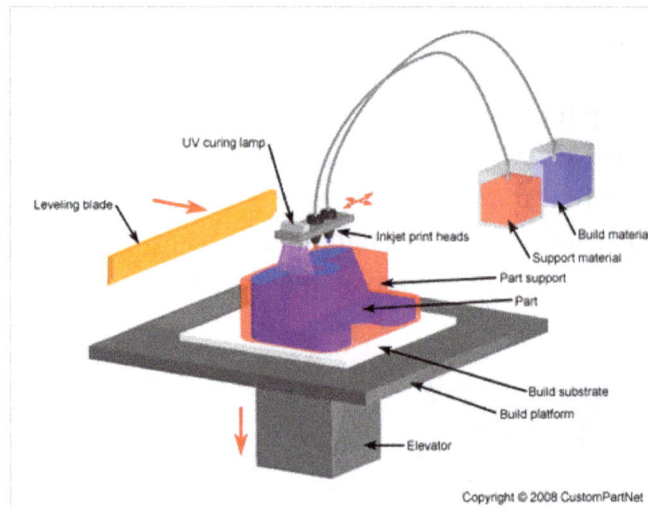

Figure 3. Schematic view of PolyJet [116].

4. Accuracy of 3D printing

Additive manufacturing plays a critical role in craniomaxillofacial surgery [49].

3D models simulate anatomy of the human body and can be extensively useful in oral and maxillofacial surgery. These models are of great value in decision making [50]. 3D models must be precise and extremely accurate in simulating head and neck anatomy to be beneficial in maxillofacial surgery. Faulty and inexact models can jeopardize diagnosis and treatment planning [16, 51]. There is limited data available about evaluation of the accuracy of 3D printed models. Inaccurate models can cause dramatic errors in treatment planning and simulations [49]. 3D printer accuracy generally depends on the accuracy of CT scans. CT is modality of choice for 3D printing purposes. While obtaining CT images, each slice thickness must be as thin as possible (1–2 mm) [30]. At present, no gold standard is introduced for measuring the accuracy of medical 3D models [49]. The accuracy of different additive manufacturing technologies is examined by researchers in maxillofacial surgery globally. The literature indicates that different techniques have different accuracy levels in reconstructing maxillofacial structures using 3D printing. As mentioned before, experiences have pointed out that SL creates 3D models with great accuracy. Average deviation of SL models varies from 0.20– 0.85 mm. Error percentage in these models is between 0.6 and 6% [17, 30, 52–54]. Peter Shih-Hsin Chang et al. investigated the accuracy of SL for modeling midface irregularities. This was done comparing distances between key landmarks on the skulls and 3D models. Average overall difference between replicas and cadaver samples was between 0.8 and 2.5 mm in all locations. They stated that SL preciseness is affected by variants in different stages of manufacturing such as data collection and transfer, product fabrication, and maintenance [38]. Preciseness and accuracy is critical in orthognathic surgery for gaining better results both esthetically and functionally. In a recent study, Shqaidef et al. evaluated the accuracy of 3D printed wafers of 10 orthognathic patients. After aligning with dental models, the absolute mean error of the wafers was 0.94 (0.09) mm. In this research, they showed error in 3D printed models is up to 1.73 mm which is considerable and will distort skeletal movements [55]. In another study, the PolyJet technique had the most precise fabrication in simulating mandibular architecture [50].

Salmi et al. assessed the accuracy of different 3D printing techniques by measuring balls attached to each 3D model. It was concluded that the PolyJet technique had the least inaccuracies [49].

Table 3 demonstrates results of different studies with accuracy measurement of 3D printed models.

Authors	Comparisons	Mean difference (%)	Measuring equipment
Salmi et al. (2013)	SLS e 3D CT (original 1. & 2. model) 3DP e 3D CT (original 1. & 2. measurement) 3DP e 3D CT (moderate) 3DP e 3D CT (worse)PolyJet e 3D CT (original 1. & 2. measurement)	0.79 0.26 & 0.80 0.320.67 0.43 & 0.69 0.440.38 0.220.55 0.370.18 0.12 & 0.18 0.13	Coordinate measuring machine and measuring balls & Pro Engineer software for 3D models
El-Katatny et al. (2010)	FDM e 3D CT skullFDM e 3D CT mandible	0.24 0.160.22 0.11	Digital caliper
Ibrahim et al. (2009)	SLS e dry mandible3DP e dry mandiblePolyJet e dry mandible	1.793.142.14	Digital caliper and test indicator attached to electric milling machine
Silva et al. (2008)	SLS e dry skull3DP e dry skull	2.102.67	Digital caliper
Nizam et al.(2006)	SL e dry skull	0.08 1.25	Digital caliper
Chang et al. (2003)	3DP e fresh skull	2.1e4.7	Dial caliper
Choi et al. (2002)	SL e dry skullSL e 3D CT skull	0.56 0.390.82 0.52	Caliper & MagicsviewSoftware for 3D model
Asaumi et al. (2001)	3D CT e dry skullSL e dry skull	2.160.63	Caliper & 3DCT images
Berry et al. (1997)	SLS e 3D CT	0.64	None reported
Barker et al. (1994)	SL e dry skull	0.6e3.6	
Ono et al. (1994)	SL e dry skull	3	
Waitzman et al. (1992)	3D CT e dry skull	0.9 (0.1e3.0)	CT images & caliper

Dawood, A., B. M. Marti, V. Sauret-Jackson and A. Darwood (2015). "3D printing in dentistry." *British dental journal* **219**(11): 521-529.

Mehra, P., J. Miner, R. D'Innocenzo and M. Nadershah (2011). "Use of 3-d stereolithographic models in oral and maxillofacial surgery." *Journal of maxillofacial and oral surgery* **10**(1): 6-13.

Salmi, M., K.-S. Paloheimo, J. Tuomi, J. Wolff and A. Mäkitie (2013). "Accuracy of medical models made by additive manufacturing (rapid manufacturing)." *Journal of Cranio-Maxillofacial Surgery* **41**(7): 603-609.

Table 3. Studies with accuracy measurement of AM models [49].

5. Clinical applications

Three-dimensional printing has been available for over three decades. Despite that, medicine has benefitted from its application recently [23–25]. As mentioned before, 3D printed models can be useful in different aspects of maxillofacial surgery such as templates, splints, tailored implants, and others [23–27]. These models can reduce surgery duration and enhance the results [10]. RP technology can become very useful for both doctor and patients in treatment planning for each patient individually [56]. Medical applications of 3D printers have expanded after recent advancements of these systems. In oral and maxillofacial surgery, 3D printing methods have been utilized for different purposes including distraction osteogenesis and treatment of craniofacial deformities [57, 58]. The following are the main applications of 3D printing technology in oral and maxillofacial surgery:

5.1. Surgical planning

Since 3D printing can distinguish traumatic and pathologic defects more effectively, it has proven to enhance diagnosis and treatment in the maxillofacial region. This feature results in precise decision making. In the aspect of pathologic lesions, 3D printing is capable of presenting spatial relationships to surrounding components [52–54, 58–63]. These important visualizations can minimize operative complications [26].

By 3D printing, surgeons can visualize the procedure and forecast the challenges to gain better results before they even start. Three-dimensional printing can produce models rapidly with acceptable accuracy and structural details to allow for better outcomes and reduced operating durations [64].

5.2. Trauma surgery

3D printers can facilitate the treatment of trauma patients with recent or delayed fractures and defects. Different fractures of maxillofacial structures can benefit from 3D printing but orbital wall fractures are the best targets for these methods [65–67]. These patients can be treated by 3D customized reconstruction of orbital wall defects with titanium mesh or sheet [68]. Before the surgery begins, titanium mesh or plate is adapted precisely on the 3D printed replica to help shortening the duration of general anesthesia [69, 70].

Complicated and detailed anatomy of the orbit makes it difficult to reconstruct orbital defects. Postoperative enophthalmos or diplopia always happens without accurate and proper reconstruction of orbital walls. Surgeons can solve these complications by using 3D printed titanium mesh using the contralateral orbital anatomy [30, 71].

Sasˇa et al. evaluated the application of custom-made implants using 3D printing system to reconstruct in blowout fractures of the orbital floor. After the surgery, average orbital volume (OV) of the affected side noticeably decreased, and OV of corrected orbit was not different compared to the unaffected side [72].

Chandan Jadhav et al. treated three patients with medial orbital wall fractures using 3D models. They used the 3D model as a template to measure and harvest bone graft from iliac crest easily and precisely, resulting in perfect adaptation and reduced operation time (**Figures 4** and **5**) [56].

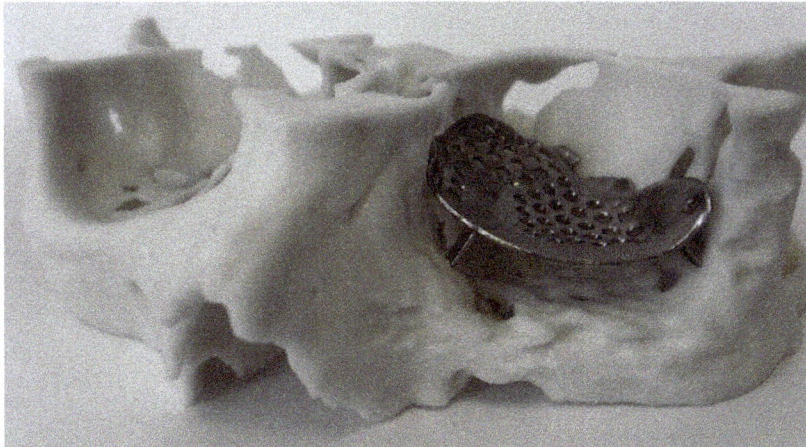

Figure 4. The rapid prototype metal orbital floor reconstruction in the orbit of the stereolithic skull reconstructed from the original CT scans [71].

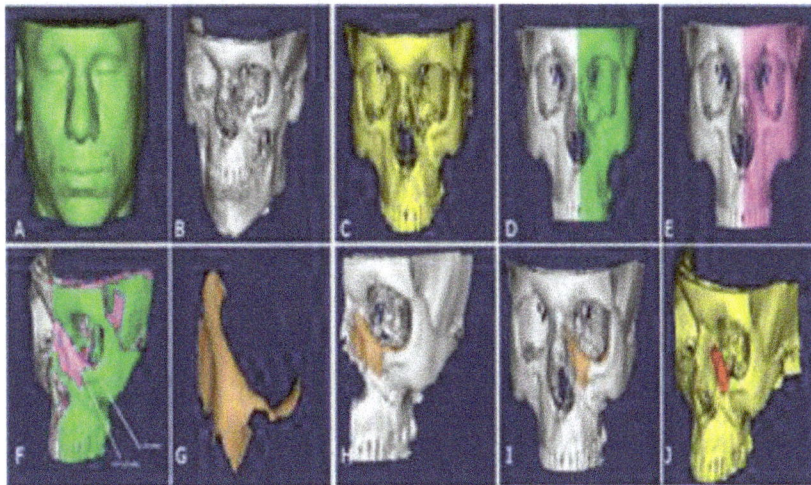

Figure 5. Treatment of orbital floor defect in a trauma patient using 3D printing technology. (a) 3D model designed based on CT scan images; (b) removal of soft tissue on differences between soft and hard tissue density; (c) removal of excess bone; (d) dividing the face into two halves from symmetry line; (e) mirroring the uninjured side on the other side; (f) comparison of the injured half and the mirrored half and finding their differences; (g) differentiation of the ideal design; (h) precise adaption on injured half; (i) correction of the design by removal of excess components; (j) final model.

5.3. Orthognathic surgery

Precise planning and decision making based on exact diagnosis is critical in the success of orthognathic surgeries [73]. As mentioned earlier, 3D printing technology shows some clinically noticeable inaccuracies for orthognathic surgery which is troublesome for ideal dental occlusion [30].

5.4. Facial prosthetics

There are reports of fabricating prosthetic nose [74, 75], ears [76, 77], eyes [78, 79], and face [80, 81], in the last 10 years. Literature indicates that better esthetic and functional outcomes are accomplished with the application of 3D printing in comparison to the traditional prosthetics (**Figure 6**) [76, 82].

Facial prosthetics fabricated with RP methods are being utilized successfully. Ancient Egyptians were the first people to apply facial prosthetics in 500 B.C [83].

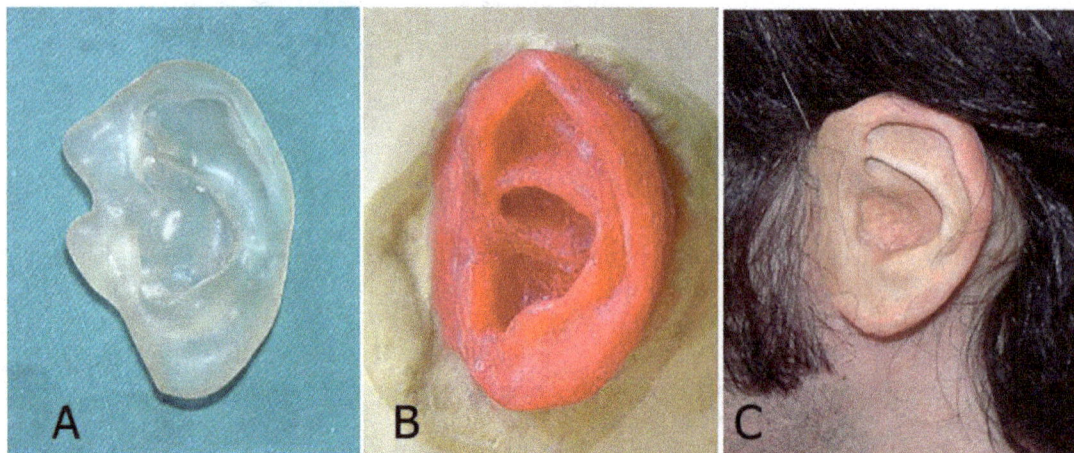

Figure 6. (a) 3D model obtained by stereolithography; (b) stereolithographic model turned into wax; (c) finished auricular prosthesis [85].

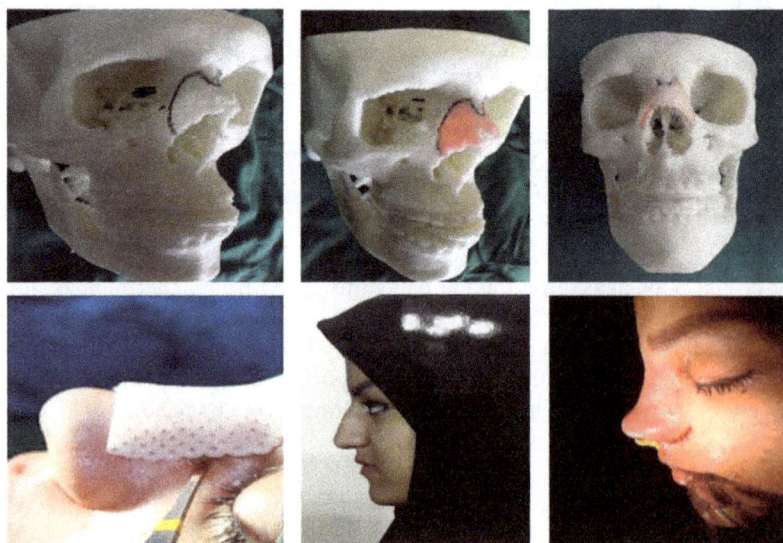

Figure 7. Application of 3D printing in lateral nasal osteotomy. (a) Planned osteotomy lines of lateral nasal osteotomy are drawn with a skin marker on the 3D model; (b) compensate the thickness of the soft tissue lining of the nose with thick wax; (c) trimming the custom-made splint on the 3D model; (d) performing the lateral nasal osteotomy in line with the surgical plan; (e) pre- and postoperative views [117].

Facial prosthetics have evolved extensively with the application of 3D printing technology. This technique allows producing replicas of facial structure within just hours [84].

Impression procedures are the common method to manufacture facial prosthetics. Longer duration of production, soft tissue distortion, and patient discomfort are the main limitations of this process. Lately, 3D printing has been utilized to produce facial prosthetics to reduce limitations of traditional procedures. Additive manufacturing technology can simplify the procedure, shorten laboratory procedures by excluding impression procedures, and model wax-ups. No doubt, 3D printing will become the modality of choice to manufacture facial prosthetics [85]. Additive manufacturing is mainly used for hard tissue reconstruction. However, it is useful in soft tissue contouring [5, 86] such as auricular reconstruction in patients using the contralateral ear (**Figure 7**) [87].

Auricular prosthesis production consists of multiple time-consuming processes demanding patient presence. These procedures are (1) impression making, (2) fabricating a wax replica, (3) manufacturing a mold, and (4) creating the prosthetic object with a suitable color. 3D printing technique simplifies and shrinks the first three steps. The process can be completed in 24–48 hours instead of a week [88].

5.5. Customized TMJ reconstruction

In the field of TMJ(Temporomandibular Joint) reconstruction, sufficient exposure and access is critical to prevent damaging many vital structures in this area. Alloplasts and allografts must be accurately placed to regain correct function of the jaw [89]. 3D printing can become useful in the treatment of TMD(Temporomandibular Joint Disorders) patients with total condylar resorption [18]. Mehra et al. treated a patient by bone grafting and TMJ prostheses using additive manufacturing. 3D printing aided in measuring exact proportions of the bone needs to be harvested [22].

5.6. Dental implants

Creation of new dental implants has benefitted from 3D printing technology [90, 91].

3D printing acts as a tool to create dental implants with complicated geometries [14].

Drilling guides are of great value to transfer implants from their planned positions. Manufacturing a drilling guide by conventional methods is time-consuming and requires multiple patient visits and extensive laboratory work. RP facilitates this with solely a single consultation prior to operation. In this session, data are gathered, and the guide is virtually built and later will be manufactured by the 3D device [92].

5.7. Complex facial reconstruction

Pathologic lesions, traumatic events, and infections are main etiologies of mandibular defects needing partial resection and bone reconstruction [93, 94]. Maintaining acceptable esthetic and functional outcomes and facial symmetry are the main goals of mandibular reconstructions. Titanium reconstruction plates are biocompatible and adaptable alloplasts for temporary reconstructions [95]. For more reliable reconstruction, autogenous bone grafts are commonly used. Complex mandibular morphology and muscular attachments moving the jaw in unfavorable positions are challenging to oral and maxillofacial surgeons in mandibular reconstructions [23]. 3D printing technology can be used in different aspects of facial reconstruction. This technology is widely used for mandibular reconstruction [96]. Better anatomical understanding, proper plate adaptation, plate pre-bending, precise bone harvesting by utilizing negative templates of the defect, reduced bone-plate distance, decreased duration of surgery, less blood loss, and shortened duration of general anesthesia are the main advantages of using additive manufacturing in mandibular reconstruction (**Figure 8**) [23, 96].

Hanasono and Skorackil indicated that 3D printing can reduce surgery duration up to 1.4 hour [97].

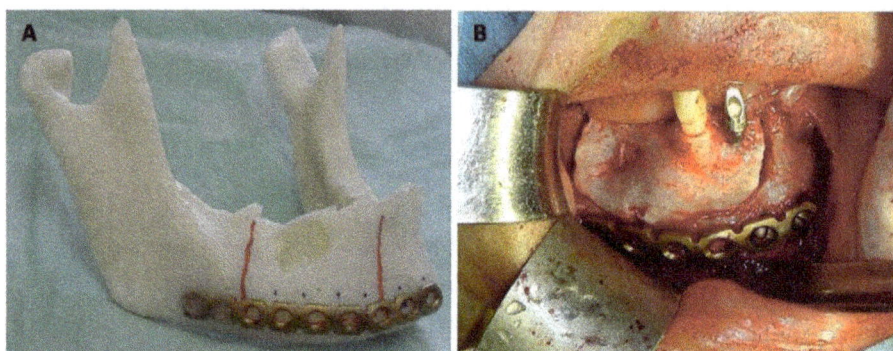

Figure 8. (a) Precontoured reconstruction plate before marginal mandibulectomy aiming to reinforce the remaining thin mandibular lower border; (b) note the anatomic alignment of the precontoured plate to the lower mandibular border [23].

6. Improvements in learning, training, and practice

6.1. Surgical education

Medical training can reform with enhancements of 3D printing technology [84].

As oral and maxillofacial surgeons, we are expected to master detailed morphology of the head and neck region and their spatial relationship. Patients and medical trainees and residents can benefit from 3D printed models [26, 98]. High maintenance charges, cultural and social complications, and formalin-related safety issues are making cadavers a limited source for medical education [99, 100].

Medical trainees can have better understanding of anatomical structure with 3D printed models.

These models allow a thorough and complete training before a surgery even begins [101, 102]. Operators can perform complicated surgeries on 3D models without any concerns and complications [103]. 3D printing also can aid in better understanding of patients' medical situation rather than a flat 2D screen [12]. Kah Heng Alexander et al. conducted a double blind randomized controlled trial to compare the success of 3D printing with human cadavers for distinguishing external cardiac anatomy. 3D printed models had significantly higher scores in comparison to the cadavers or combined groups [98]. With the enhancement of new materials, 3D printed models will be more accurate in the future [104–106].

6.2. Patient education

Fulfilling patient expectations is critical to have successful surgical outcomes. Surgeon-patient professional relationship can be simplified using 3D printing. In preoperative consultations, patients can understand surgical details, different results, and potential obstacles. Therefore, 3D printed models can aid gaining informed consent. [103]. CT/MRI scans that we use today to explain the procedure for the patients are usually hard to understand for uneducated patients. Patients mostly do not comprehend the situation.

Literature has shown that 3D printed models result in better training of both patients and medical trainees [26, 107, 108]. Also having in-office preoperative and postoperative 3D printed models of specific surgeries can help patients justify their expectations [26].

Patients' families can also benefit from additive manufacturing since they might have positive impacts on patient satisfaction. These models could be utilized to form a library for future educational goals [109].

7. Prospective visions

Three-dimensional printers are a new and emerging technology with the ability to manufacture physical objects from digital files. Decreasing hardware costs have made this technology affordable for use in the office setting [26]. 3D printing technology enables more effective patient consultations, increases diagnostic quality, improves surgical planning, acts as an orientation aid during surgical procedures, and manufactures guiding template segmental resections. In the future, additive manufacturing might be capable of organ bio-printing [30]. Surgery is a practical art! The surgeon often uses direct physical intervention in the treatment of patients. Surgical procedures must be accurately planned for each patient individually to minimize complications and increase benefits. In oral and maxillofacial surgery, potential uses extend to surgical planning, education, and prosthetic device design and development. RP is not utilized in conventional clinical applications but can revolutionize oral and maxillofacial surgery in the future [26]. To clarify and understand what is the best prediction for the future of the technology itself, production time of objects and costs should also be considered. Different researchers have indicated that they have found 3D printing a cost-effective technology [110–112]. However, some other investigators have doubted efficiency and price of RP [113]. 3D printed replicas are considered to be more precise and cost-effective for patients and trainee education compared to other techniques [114]. This method also eliminates the need for animal studies [64]. 3D printing technology is here to improve our lifestyle and health care in the twenty-first century [103].

Author details

Seied Omid Keyhan[1], Sina Ghanean[2*], Alireza Navabazam[2], Arash Khojasteh[3] and Mohammad Hosein Amirzade Iranaq[4]

*Address all correspondence to: sinasin@gmail.com

1 Department of Oral and Maxillofacial Surgery, Shahid Sadoughi & Shahid Beheshti University of Medical Sciences, Dental Research Center, Yazd-Tehran, Iran

2 Department of Oral and Maxillofacial Surgery, Shahid Sadoughi University of Medical Sciences, Yazd, Iran

3 Department of Oral and Maxillofacial Surgery, Shahid Beheshti University of Medical Sciences, Tehran, Iran. Dean, School of Advanced Technologies in Medicine, Tehran, Iran

4 Student Research Committee, Shahid Sadoughi University of Medical Sciences, Yazd, Iran

References

[1] Gibbs DM, Vaezi M, Yang S, Oreffo RO. Hope versus hype: what can additive manufacturing realistically offer trauma and orthopedic surgery? Regenerative Medicine. 2014;9(4):535–49.

[2] Canstein C, Cachot P, Faust A, Stalder A, Bock J, Frydrychowicz A, et al. 3D MR flow analysis in realistic rapid-prototyping model systems of the thoracic aorta: comparison with in vivo data and computational fluid dynamics in identical vessel geometries. Magnetic Resonance in Medicine. 2008;59(3):535–46.

[3] Müller A, Krishnan KG, Uhl E, Mast G. The application of rapid prototyping techniques in cranial reconstruction and preoperative planning in neurosurgery. Journal of Craniofacial Surgery. 2003;14(6):899–914.

[4] Hoy MB. 3D printing: making things at the library. Medical Reference Services Quarterly. 2013;32(1):93–9.

[5] Rengier F, Mehndiratta A, von Tengg-Kobligk H, Zechmann CM, Unterhinninghofen R, Kauczor H-U, et al. 3D printing based on imaging data: review of medical applications. International Journal of Computer Assisted Radiology and Surgery. 2010;5(4): 335–41.

[6] Chae MP, Rozen WM, McMenamin PG, Findlay MW, Spychal RT, Hunter-Smith DJ. Emerging applications of bedside 3D printing in plastic surgery. Frontiers in Surgery. 2015;2.

[7] Mertz L. New world of 3-d printing offers "completely new ways of thinking": q&a with author, engineer, and 3-d printing expert hod lipson. IEEE Pulse. 2013;4(6):12–4.

[8] Ibrahim AM, Jose RR, Rabie AN, Gerstle TL, Lee BT, Lin SJ. Three-dimensional printing in developing countries. Plastic and Reconstructive Surgery Global Open. 2015;3(7).

[9] Chan HH, Siewerdsen JH, Vescan A, Daly MJ, Prisman E, Irish JC. 3D rapid prototyping for otolaryngology—head and neck surgery: applications in image-guidance, surgical simulation and patient-specific modeling. PLoS One. 2015;10(9):e0136370.

[10] Mendez BM, Chiodo MV, Patel PA. Customized "In-Office" three-dimensional printing for virtual surgical planning in craniofacial surgery. Journal of Craniofacial Surgery. 2015;26(5):1584–6.

[11] Cunningham LL, Madsen MJ, Peterson G. Stereolithographic modeling technology applied to tumor resection. Journal of Oral and Maxillofacial Surgery. 2005;63(6):873–8.

[12] AlAli AB, Griffin MF, Butler PE. Three-dimensional printing surgical applications. Eplasty. 2015;15.

[13] Hull CW. Apparatus for production of three-dimensional objects by stereolithography. Google Patents; 1986.

[14] Dawood A, Marti BM, Sauret-Jackson V, Darwood A. 3D printing in dentistry. British Dental Journal. 2015;219(11):521–9.

[15] Brix F, Hebbinghaus D, Meyer W. Verfahren und Vorrichtung für den Modellbau im Rahmen der orthopädischen und traumatologischen Operationsplanung. Röntgenpraxis. 1985;38:290–2.

[16] Sinn DP, Cillo Jr JE, Miles BA. Stereolithography for craniofacial surgery. Journal of Craniofacial Surgery. 2006;17(5):869–75.

[17] Mankovich NJ, Cheeseman AM, Stoker NG. The display of three-dimensional anatomy with stereolithographic models. Journal of Digital Imaging. 1990;3(3):200–3.

[18] Suomalainen A, Stoor P, Mesimäki K, Kontio RK. Rapid prototyping modelling in oral and maxillofacial surgery: a two year retrospective study. Journal of Clinical and Experimental Dentistry. 2015;7(5):e605.

[19] Barker T, Earwaker W, Lisle D. Accuracy of stereolithographic models of human anatomy. Australasian Radiology. 1994;38(2):106–11.

[20] Frühwald J, Schicho KA, Figl M, Benesch T, Watzinger F, Kainberger F. Accuracy of craniofacial measurements: computed tomography and three-dimensional computed tomography compared with stereolithographic models. Journal of Craniofacial Surgery. 2008;19(1):22–6.

[21] Mazzoli A, Germani M, Moriconi G. Application of optical digitizing techniques to evaluate the shape accuracy of anatomical models derived from computed tomography data. Journal of Oral and Maxillofacial Surgery. 2007;65(7):1410–8.

[22] Mehra P, Miner J, D'Innocenzo R, Nadershah M. Use of 3-d stereolithographic models in oral and maxillofacial surgery. Journal of Maxillofacial and Oral Surgery. 2011;10(1): 6–13.

[23] Cohen A, Laviv A, Berman P, Nashef R, Abu-Tair J. Mandibular reconstruction using stereolithographic 3-dimensional printing modeling technology. Oral Surgery, Oral Medicine, Oral Pathology, Oral Radiology, and Endodontology. 2009;108(5):661–6.

[24] Mazzoni S, Marchetti C, Sgarzani R, Cipriani R, Scotti R, Ciocca L. Prosthetically guided maxillofacial surgery: evaluation of the accuracy of a surgical guide and custom-made bone plate in oncology patients after mandibular reconstruction. Plastic and Reconstructive Surgery. 2013;131(6):1376–85.

[25] Eppley BL, Sadove AM. Computer-generated patient models for reconstruction of cranial and facial deformities. Journal of Craniofacial Surgery. 1998;9(6):548–56.

[26] Gerstle TL, Ibrahim AM, Kim PS, Lee BT, Lin SJ. A plastic surgery application in evolution: three-dimensional printing. Plastic and Reconstructive Surgery. 2014;133(2): 446–51.

[27] Chopra K, Gastman BR, Manson PN. Stereolithographic modeling in reconstructive surgery of the craniofacial skeleton after tumor resection. Plastic and Reconstructive Surgery. 2012;129(4):743e–5e.

[28] Melchels FP, Feijen J, Grijpma DW. A review on stereolithography and its applications in biomedical engineering. Biomaterials. 2010;31(24):6121–30.

[29] Yan X, Gu P. A review of rapid prototyping technologies and systems. Computer-Aided Design. 1996;28(4):307–18.

[30] Choi JW, Kim N. Clinical application of three-dimensional printing technology in craniofacial plastic surgery. Archives of Plastic Surgery. 2015;42(3):267–77.

[31] Dowler C. Automatic model building cuts design time, costs. Plastics Engineering. 1989;45(4):43–5.

[32] Fisher JP, Dean D, Mikos AG. Photocrosslinking characteristics and mechanical properties of diethyl fumarate/poly (propylene fumarate) biomaterials. Biomaterials. 2002;23(22):4333–43.

[33] Billiet T, Vandenhaute M, Schelfhout J, Van Vlierberghe S, Dubruel P. A review of trends and limitations in hydrogel-rapid prototyping for tissue engineering. Biomaterials. 2012;33(26):6020–41.

[34] Rozen WM, Ting JW, Leung M, Wu T, Ying D, Leong J. Advancing image-guided surgery in microvascular mandibular reconstruction: combining bony and vascular

imaging with computed tomography–guided stereolithographic bone modeling. Plastic and Reconstructive Surgery. 2012;130(1):227e–9e.

[35] Rozen WM, Ting JW, Baillieu C, Leong J. Stereolithographic modeling of the deep circumflex iliac artery and its vascular branching: a further advance in computed tomography–guided flap planning. Plastic and Reconstructive Surgery. 2012;130(2): 380e–2e.

[36] Hannen E. Recreating the original contour in tumor deformed mandibles for plate adapting. International Journal of Oral and Maxillofacial Surgery. 2006;35(2):183–5.

[37] Ono I, Gunji H, Suda K, Kaneko F. Method for preparing an exact-size model using helical volume scan computed tomography. Plastic and Reconstructive Surgery. 1994;93(7):1363.

[38] Chang PS-H, Parker TH, Patrick CW, Miller MJ. The accuracy of stereolithography in planning craniofacial bone replacement. Journal of Craniofacial Surgery. 2003;14(2): 164–70.

[39] Choi J-Y, Choi J-H, Kim N-K, Kim Y, Lee J-K, Kim M-K, et al. Analysis of errors in medical rapid prototyping models. International Journal of Oral and Maxillofacial Surgery. 2002;31(1):23–32.

[40] Chia HN, Wu BM. Recent advances in 3D printing of biomaterials. Journal of Biological Engineering. 2015;9(1):4.

[41] Herlin C, Koppe M, Béziat J-L, Gleizal A. Rapid prototyping in craniofacial surgery: using a positioning guide after zygomatic osteotomy–a case report. Journal of Cranio-Maxillofacial Surgery. 2011;39(5):376–9.

[42] Zhang X, Jiang X, Sun C. Micro-stereolithography of polymeric and ceramic micro-structures. Sensors and Actuators A: Physical. 1999;77(2):149–56.

[43] Krishnan S, Dawood A, Richards R, Henckel J, Hart A. A review of rapid prototyped surgical guides for patient-specific total knee replacement. Journal of Bone & Joint Surgery, British Volume. 2012;94(11):1457–61.

[44] Fortin T, Champleboux G, Lormée J, Coudert JL. Precise dental implant placement in bone using surgical guides in conjunction with medical imaging techniques. Journal of Oral Implantology. 2000;26(4):300–3.

[45] Flügge TV, Nelson K, Schmelzeisen R, Metzger MC. Three-dimensional plotting and printing of an implant drilling guide: simplifying guided implant surgery. Journal of Oral and Maxillofacial Surgery. 2013;71(8):1340–6.

[46] Dikovsky D, Napadensky E. Three-dimensional printing process for producing a self-destructible temporary structure. Google Patents; 2013.

[47] Ohtani T, Kusumoto N, Wakabayashi K, Yamada S, Nakamura T, Kumazawa Y, et al. Application of haptic device to implant dentistry-accuracy verification of drilling into a pig bone. Dental Materials Journal. 2009;28(1):75–81.

[48] Almquist TA, Smalley DR. Thermal stereolithography. Google Patents; 1996.

[49] Salmi M, Paloheimo K-S, Tuomi J, Wolff J, Mäkitie A. Accuracy of medical models made by additive manufacturing (rapid manufacturing). Journal of Cranio-Maxillofacial Surgery. 2013;41(7):603–9.

[50] Silva DN, De Oliveira MG, Meurer E, Meurer MI, da Silva JVL, Santa-Bárbara A. Dimensional error in selective laser sintering and 3D-printing of models for cranio-maxillary anatomy reconstruction. Journal of Cranio-Maxillofacial Surgery. 2008;36(8): 443–9.

[51] Lethaus B, Poort L, Böckmann R, Smeets R, Tolba R, Kessler P. Additive manufacturing for microvascular reconstruction of the mandible in 20 patients. Journal of Cranio-Maxillofacial Surgery. 2012;40(1):43–6.

[52] Klimek L, Klein H, Schneider W, Mösges R, Schmelzer B, Voy E. Stereolithographic modelling for reconstructive head surgery. Acta Oto-rhino-laryngologica Belgica. 1992;47(3):329–34.

[53] Swaelens B, Kruth J-P, editors. Medical applications of rapid prototyping techniques. Proceedings of the 2nd European Conference on Rapid Prototyping; 1993.

[54] Arvier J, Barker T, Yau Y, D'Urso P, Atkinson R, McDermant G. Maxillofacial biomodelling. British Journal of Oral and Maxillofacial Surgery. 1994;32(5):276–83.

[55] Shqaidef A, Ayoub AF, Khambay BS. How accurate are rapid prototyped (RP) final orthognathic surgical wafers? A pilot study. British Journal of Oral and Maxillofacial Surgery. 2014;52(7):609–14.

[56] Ata N. Complete mulberry hypertrophy and conchachoanal polyp of inferior turbinate. Journal of Craniofacial Surgery. 2015;26(8):e799.

[57] Gateno J, Xia J, Teichgraeber JF, Rosen A, Hultgren B, Vadnais T. The precision of computer-generated surgical splints. Journal of Oral and Maxillofacial Surgery. 2003;61(7):814–7.

[58] Poukens J, Haex J, Riediger D. The use of rapid prototyping in the preoperative planning of distraction osteogenesis of the cranio-maxillofacial skeleton. Computer Aided Surgery. 2003;8(3):146–54.

[59] Dittmann W, Bill J, Wittenberg G, Reuther J, Roosen K. Stereolithography as a new method of reconstructive surgical planning in complex osseous defects of the cranial base. Technical note. Zentralblatt für Neurochirurgie. 1994;55(4):209.

[60] Bill JS, Reuther JF, Dittmann W, Kübler N, Meier JL, Pistner H, et al. Stereolithography in oral and maxillofacial operation planning. International Journal of Oral and Maxillofacial Surgery. 1995;24(1):98–103.

[61] Stoker NG, Mankovich NJ, Valentino D. Stereolithographic models for surgical planning: preliminary report. Journal of Oral and Maxillofacial Surgery. 1992;50(5):466–71.

[62] Jacobs PF. Stereolithography and other RP&M technologies: from rapid prototyping to rapid tooling. Society of Manufacturing Engineers; 1995.

[63] Paul F. Rapid prototyping and manufacturing, fundamentals of stereolithography. SME, Dearborn, MI; 1992;8:135–41.

[64] Klein GT, Lu Y, Wang MY. 3D printing and neurosurgery—ready for prime time? World neurosurgery. 2013;80(3):233–5.

[65] Olszewski R, Tranduy K, Reychler H. Innovative procedure for computer-assisted genioplasty: three-dimensional cephalometry, rapid-prototyping model and surgical splint. International Journal of Oral and Maxillofacial Surgery. 2010;39(7):721–4.

[66] Michalski MH, Ross JS. The shape of things to come: 3D printing in medicine. JAMA. 2014;312(21):2213–4.

[67] Fullerton JN, Frodsham GC, Day RM. 3D printing for the many, not the few. Nature Biotechnology. 2014;32(11):1086–7.

[68] Mustafa S, Evans P, Bocca A, Patton D, Sugar A, Baxter P. Customized titanium reconstruction of post-traumatic orbital wall defects: a review of 22 cases. International Journal of Oral and Maxillofacial Surgery. 2011;40(12):1357–62.

[69] Kozakiewicz M, Elgalal M, Piotr L, Broniarczyk-Loba A, Stefanczyk L. Treatment with individual orbital wall implants in humans–1-year ophthalmologic evaluation. Journal of Cranio-Maxillofacial Surgery. 2011;39(1):30–6.

[70] Kozakiewicz M, Elgalal M, Loba P, Komuński P, Arkuszewski P, Broniarczyk-Loba A, et al. Clinical application of 3D pre-bent titanium implants for orbital floor fractures. Journal of Cranio-Maxillofacial Surgery. 2009;37(4):229–34.

[71] Wolff J, Sándor GK, Pyysalo M, Miettinen A, Koivumäki A-V, Kainulainen VT. Late reconstruction of orbital and naso-orbital deformities. Oral and Maxillofacial Surgery Clinics of North America. 2013;25(4):683–95.

[72] Tabakovic SZ, Konstantinovic VS, Radosavljevic R, Movrin D, Hadžistevic M, Hatab N. Application of computer-aided designing and rapid prototyping technologies in reconstruction of blowout fractures of the orbital floor. Journal of Craniofacial Surgery. 2015;26(5):1558–63.

[73] Metzger MC, Hohlweg-Majert B, Schwarz U, Teschner M, Hammer B, Schmelzeisen R. Manufacturing splints for orthognathic surgery using a three-dimensional printer. Oral

Surgery, Oral Medicine, Oral Pathology, Oral Radiology, and Endodontology. 2008;105(2):e1–7.

[74] Wu G, Zhou B, Bi Y, Zhao Y. Selective laser sintering technology for customized fabrication of facial prostheses. The Journal of Prosthetic Dentistry. 2008;100(1):56–60.

[75] Ciocca L, De Crescenzio F, Fantini M, Scotti R. Rehabilitation of the nose using CAD/CAM and rapid prototyping technology after ablative surgery of squamous cell carcinoma: a pilot clinical report. The International Journal of Oral & Maxillofacial Implants. 2009;25(4):808–12.

[76] Sykes LM, Parrott AM, Owen CP, Snaddon DR. Applications of rapid prototyping technology in maxillofacial prosthetics. The International Journal of Prosthodontics. 2003;17(4):454–9.

[77] Ciocca L, De Crescenzio F, Fantini M, Scotti R. CAD/CAM bilateral ear prostheses construction for Treacher Collins syndrome patients using laser scanning and rapid prototyping. Computer Methods in Biomechanics and Biomedical Engineering. 2010;13(3):379–86.

[78] Xie P, Hu Z, Zhang X, Li X, Gao Z, Yuan D, et al. Application of 3-dimensional printing technology to construct an eye model for fundus viewing study. 2014.

[79] Ciocca L, Scotti R. Oculo-facial rehabilitation after facial cancer removal: updated CAD/CAM procedures. A pilot study. Prosthetics and Orthotics International. 2013:0309364613512368.

[80] Fantini M, De Crescenzio F, Ciocca L. Design and rapid manufacturing of anatomical prosthesis for facial rehabilitation. International Journal on Interactive Design and Manufacturing (IJIDeM). 2013;7(1):51–62.

[81] Tsuji M, Noguchi N, Ihara K, Yamashita Y, Shikimori M, Goto M. Fabrication of a maxillofacial prosthesis using a computer-aided design and manufacturing system. Journal of Prosthodontics. 2004;13(3):179–83.

[82] Karayazgan-Saracoglu B, Gunay Y, Atay A. Fabrication of an auricular prosthesis using computed tomography and rapid prototyping technique. Journal of Craniofacial Surgery. 2009;20(4):1169–72.

[83] Reisberg DJ, Habakuk SW. A history of facial and ocular prosthetics. Advances in Ophthalmic Plastic and Reconstructive Surgery. 1989;8:11–24.

[84] Bauermeister AJ, Zuriarrain A, Newman MI. Three-dimensional printing in plastic and reconstructive surgery: a systematic review. Annals of Plastic Surgery. 2015.

[85] Karatas MO, Cifter ED, Ozenen DO, Balik A, Tuncer EB. Manufacturing implant supported auricular prostheses by rapid prototyping techniques. European Journal of Dentistry. 2011;5(4):472.

[86] Lindsay RW, Herberg M, Liacouras P. The use of three-dimensional digital technology and additive manufacturing to create templates for soft-tissue reconstruction. Plastic and Reconstructive Surgery. 2012;130(4):630e–2e.

[87] Subburaj K, Nair C, Rajesh S, Meshram S, Ravi B. Rapid development of auricular prosthesis using CAD and rapid prototyping technologies. International Journal of Oral and Maxillofacial Surgery. 2007;36(10):938–43.

[88] Liacouras P, Garnes J, Roman N, Petrich A, Grant GT. Designing and manufacturing an auricular prosthesis using computed tomography, 3-dimensional photographic imaging, and additive manufacturing: a clinical report. The Journal of Prosthetic Dentistry. 2011;105(2):78–82.

[89] Levine JP, Patel A, Saadeh PB, Hirsch DL. Computer-aided design and manufacturing in craniomaxillofacial surgery: the new state of the art. Journal of Craniofacial Surgery. 2012;23(1):288–93.

[90] Chen J, Zhang Z, Chen X, Zhang C, Zhang G, Xu Z. Design and manufacture of customized dental implants by using reverse engineering and selective laser melting technology. The Journal of Prosthetic Dentistry. 2014;112(5):1088–95. e1.

[91] Xiong Y, Qian C, Sun J. Fabrication of porous titanium implants by three-dimensional printing and sintering at different temperatures. Dental Materials Journal. 2012;31(5): 815–20.

[92] Habibovic P, Gbureck U, Doillon CJ, Bassett DC, van Blitterswijk CA, Barralet JE. Osteoconduction and osteoinduction of low-temperature 3D printed bioceramic implants. Biomaterials. 2008;29(7):944–53.

[93] Chang Y-M, Shen Y-F, Lin H-N, Tsai AH-Y, Tsai C-Y, Wei F-C. Total reconstruction and rehabilitation with vascularized fibula graft and osseointegrated teeth implantation after segmental mandibulectomy for fibrous dysplasia. Plastic and Reconstructive Surgery. 2004;113(4):1205–8.

[94] Chana JS, Chang Y-M, Wei F-C, Shen Y-F, Chan C-P, Lin H-N, et al. Segmental mandibulectomy and immediate free fibula osteoseptocutaneous flap reconstruction with endosteal implants: an ideal treatment method for mandibular ameloblastoma. Plastic and Reconstructive Surgery. 2004;113(1):80–7.

[95] Futran ND, Urken ML, Buchbinder D, Moscoso JF, Biller HF. Rigid fixation of vascularized bone grafts in mandibular reconstruction. Archives of Otolaryngology–Head & Neck Surgery. 1995;121(1):70–6.

[96] Fowell C, Edmondson S, Martin T, Praveen P. Rapid prototyping and patient-specific pre-contoured reconstruction plate for comminuted fractures of the mandible. British Journal of Oral and Maxillofacial Surgery. 2015;53(10):1035–7.

[97] Hanasono M, Skoracki R. 117B: improving the speed and accuracy of mandibular reconstruction using preoperative virtual planning and rapid prototype modeling. Plastic and Reconstructive Surgery. 2010;125(6):80.

[98] Lim KHA, Loo ZY, Goldie SJ, Adams JW, McMenamin PG. Use of 3D printed models in medical education: a randomized control trial comparing 3D prints versus cadaveric materials for learning external cardiac anatomy. Anatomical Sciences Education. 2015.

[99] McMenamin PG, Quayle MR, McHenry CR, Adams JW. The production of anatomical teaching resources using three-dimensional (3D) printing technology. Anatomical Sciences Education. 2014;7(6):479–86.

[100] Lambrecht JT, Berndt D, Schumacher R, Zehnder M. Generation of three-dimensional prototype models based on cone beam computed tomography. International Journal of Computer Assisted Radiology and Surgery. 2009;4(2):175–80.

[101] Kalejs M, von Segesser LK. Rapid prototyping of compliant human aortic roots for assessment of valved stents. Interactive Cardiovascular and Thoracic Surgery. 2009;8(2):182–6.

[102] Armillotta A, Bonhoeffer P, Dubini G, Ferragina S, Migliavacca F, Sala G, et al. Use of rapid prototyping models in the planning of percutaneous pulmonary valved stent implantation. Proceedings of the Institution of Mechanical Engineers, Part H: Journal of Engineering in Medicine. 2007;221(4):407–16.

[103] Malik HH, Darwood AR, Shaunak S, Kulatilake P, Abdulrahman A, Mulki O, et al. Three-dimensional printing in surgery: a review of current surgical applications. Journal of Surgical Research. 2015;199(2):512–22.

[104] Waran V, Narayanan V, Karuppiah R, Owen SL, Aziz T. Utility of multimaterial 3D printers in creating models with pathological entities to enhance the training experience of neurosurgeons: technical note. Journal of neurosurgery. 2014;120(2):489–92.

[105] Biglino G, Verschueren P, Zegels R, Taylor AM, Schievano S. Rapid prototyping compliant arterial phantoms for in-vitro studies and device testing. Journal of Cardio-vascular Magnetic Resonance. 2013;15(2):1–7.

[106] Mashiko T, Otani K, Kawano R, Konno T, Kaneko N, Ito Y, et al. Development of three-dimensional hollow elastic model for cerebral aneurysm clipping simulation enabling rapid and low cost prototyping. World Neurosurgery. 2013.

[107] Way TP, Barner KE. Automatic visual to tactile translation. II. Evaluation of the TACTile image creation system. IEEE Transactions on Rehabilitation Engineering. 1997;5(1):95–105.

[108] Suzuki M, Ogawa Y, Kawano A, Hagiwara A, Yamaguchi H, Ono H. Rapid prototyping of temporal bone for surgical training and medical education. Acta Oto-laryngologica. 2004;124(4):400–2.

[109] Niikura T, Sugimoto M, Lee SY, Sakai Y, Nishida K, Kuroda R, et al. Tactile surgical navigation system for complex acetabular fracture surgery. Orthopedics (Online). 2014;37(4):237.

[110] Duan B, Hockaday LA, Kang KH, Butcher JT. 3D bioprinting of heterogeneous aortic valve conduits with alginate/gelatin hydrogels. Journal of Biomedical Materials Research Part A. 2013;101(5):1255–64.

[111] Dean D, Min K-J, Bond A. Computer aided design of large-format prefabricated cranial plates. Journal of Craniofacial Surgery. 2003;14(6):819–32.

[112] Condino S, Carbone M, Ferrari V, Faggioni L, Peri A, Ferrari M, et al. How to build patient-specific synthetic abdominal anatomies. An innovative approach from physical toward hybrid surgical simulators. The International Journal of Medical Robotics and Computer Assisted Surgery. 2011;7(2):202–13.

[113] Jirman R, Horák Z, Mazánek J, Řezníček J. Individual replacement of the frontal bone defect: case report. Prague Medical Report. 2009;110:79–84.

[114] Turney BW. A new model with an anatomically accurate human renal collecting system for training in fluoroscopy-guided percutaneous nephrolithotomy access. Journal of Endourology. 2014;28(3):360–3.

[115] van Noort R, The future of dental devices is digital. Dental Materials. 2012;28(1):3–12.

[116] CustomPartNet. 2009 [cited 2016 21 Jan]; Available from: http://www.custompart-net.com/wu/jetted-photopolymer.

[117] Keyhan SO. Customized lateral nasal osteotomy guide: three-dimensional printer assisted fabrication. Triple R. 2016;1(1):30–1.

6

Anesthesia and Sedation

Jeffrey A. Elo and Ho-Hyun Sun

Abstract

Anxiety control and patient comfort are integral components of everyday oral and maxillofacial surgery (OMFS) practice. Moderate sedation, deep sedation (DS), and general anesthesia (GA) have been successfully administered by and in the offices of oral and maxillofacial surgeons (OMSs) and their anesthesia teams for more than 50 years. The goal of moderate sedation, DS, or GA in the OMFS office is to establish an environment in which patients are comfortable and cooperative while allowing the surgeon to safely perform the operation. This requires meticulous care in which the practitioner balances the depth of sedation and level of responsiveness while maintaining a patent airway, proper and adequate ventilation, and optimal cardiovascular hemodynamics. The record of safety among OMSs with this form of outpatient anesthesia is exemplary. The impressive morbidity and mortality statistics support the concept that the OMFS anesthesia team model is a safe, efficient, and cost-effective model for office-based ambulatory surgical-anesthesia care. Safe anesthesia practice depends on various items, including goals of anesthesia, selecting the proper patient, anesthetic technique utilized, drug regimen selection, monitoring, anesthetic team (staff and anesthesia provider) training, and the team's preparedness to handle unanticipated complications and medical/anesthetic emergencies.

Keywords: general anesthesia, pediatric anesthesia, levels of sedation, anesthetic agents, local anesthetics

1. Introduction

Moderate sedation, deep sedation, and general anesthesia have been successfully and safely administered by and in the offices of oral and maxillofacial surgeons (OMSs) and their anesthesia teams for more than 50 years. [1–5]The goal of moderate sedation, deep sedation (DS), or general anesthesia (GA) in the oral and maxillofacial surgery (OMFS) office is to establish a safe environment in which the patient is comfortable and cooperative while allowing the surgeon to safely perform the indicated operation. This requires meticulous care in which the practitioner balances the patient's depth of sedation andlevel of responsiveness while maintaining a patent airway, proper and adequate ventilation,andoptimalcardiovascular hemodynamics. Several recent nationwide morbidity studies in the United States have demonstrated that these techniques are safe when used by OMSs who have completed an accredited OMFS residency program with formaltraininginanesthesiology. The impressivemorbidityandmortality statistics support the concept that the OMFS anesthesia team model is a safe, efficient, and cost-effective model for office-based ambulatory surgical-anesthesia care.

A preanesthetic patient assessment is a critical component of an OMS' practice. The standardization of the method of evaluating and documenting a patient's medical history and physical examination findings, as well as any pertinent diagnostic tests (laboratory and radiographic), isessentialtoformulatinganaccuratediagnosisanddevelopinganeffectiveanesthetictreatment plan. A comprehensive evaluation provides the basis for determining the surgical and anesthetic risk of each patient, and minimizes perioperative morbidity and complications associated with comorbid systemic health conditions. It is important to note that many comorbid medical conditions require consideration by the OMS. However, as each OMS has been trained during his/her surgical residency to complete a thorough pre-operative patient assessment, this chapter is not intended to describe the steps in how to perform an assessment; rather it will attempt to organize its process.

The processes described here establish a foundation for patient assessment and management as described in the American Association of Oral and Maxillofacial Surgeons' (AAOMS) Parameters of Care—2012 (AAOMS ParCare 2012) [9]. Specific diagnostic techniques and physical assessment protocols are purposely not defined, as it is not the authors' intent to dictate the methods for performing a patient assessment. The OMS has the freedom and ability to complete a patient assessment based on his/her training, the clinical circumstances of the patient, and the institutional standards under which the OMS practices.

The OMS is responsible for an initial history and physical examination necessary to determine the risk factors associated with the management of each patient. In some circumstances, the patient's primary care medical doctor may perform the history and physical examination, but it is ultimately the responsibility of the OMS to review such information and to ascertain whether it is complete to his/her level of satisfaction or whether further assessment and/or laboratory studies are indicated based on the specific patient and planned procedure. In cases when another health care provider (such as a primary care physician, cardiologist, or pediatrician) assesses the patient preoperatively, the OMS must ensure that the documented assessment also meets the parameters set forth in the AAOMS ParCare 2012 [9] The OMS is solely responsible for the final risk assessment of the patient and, ultimately, the decision to perform or not perform the surgical procedure. No other provider may assume this responsibility.

1.1. American Society of Anesthesiologists (ASA) Physical Status Patient Classification System

ASA class I	A normal healthy patient
ASA class II	A patient with mild systemic disease
ASA class III	A patient with severe systemic disease
ASA class IV	A patient with severe systemic disease that is a constant threat to life
ASA class V	A moribund patient who is not expected to survive without an operation
ASA class VI	A declared brain-dead patient whose organs are being removed for donor purposes

*Note: If a surgical procedure is performed emergently, an "E" is added to the previously defined ASA classification.

Table 1. American Society of Anesthesiologists Physical Status Patient Classification System

On the basis of a thorough patient assessment, an ASA physical status should be assigned to all surgical patients according to the guidelines set forth by the ASA (**Table 1**).

1.2. Preoperative fasting guidelines

Every healthy patient without a risk of gastroparesis who will undergo a sedation or general anesthetic procedure should maintain a "nothing per mouth" (NPO) status (**Table 2**). The ASA [10] recommends a 2-h fasting period of clear liquids for all patients. The ASA recommends a fasting period for breast milk of 4 h and for infant formula or nonhuman milk of 6 h for neonates and infants. For solid foods in most adult patients, the ASA recommends fasting periods of at least 6 h (light meal such as toast and clear liquid) or 8 h (fatty or fried foods or meat). For infants and children, the fasting period for solids should be at least 6 h.

Ingested material	Minimum fasting period
Clear liquids	2 h
Breast milk	4 h
Infant formula	6 h
Nonhuman milk	6 h
Light meal	6 h
Fatty meal	8 h

Table 2. American Society of Anesthesiologists Fasting Guidelines [10]

The preoperative use of gastric stimulants, gastric acid secretion blockers (histamine H_2 receptor antagonist agents), antacids, antiemetic agents, and/or anticholinergic medications (to decrease the risk of pulmonary aspiration) is not routinely recommended [10] Their use should be based on the individual patient assessment.

1.3. Discharge criteria

All patients who have undergone outpatient surgery using moderate sedation, DS, or GA must meet minimal criteria to permit safe discharge from the OMFS office or outpatient surgical facility. Such criteria may include either the use of an Aldrete Score (**Table 3**), Post-Anesthesia Discharge Scoring System (PADSS or modified PADSS), or another equivalent. The patient must arrive at the office or surgical facility with a responsible adult escort for discharge after surgery and anesthesia.

Criteria	Points
Oxygenation	
$SpO_2 > 92\%$ on room air	2
$SpO_2 > 90\%$ on oxygen	1
$SpO_2 < 90\%$ on oxygen	0
Respiration	
Breathes deeply and coughs freely	2
Dyspneic, shallow, or limited breathing	1
Apnea	0
Circulation	
BP ± 20% of normal	2
BP ± 20–50% of normal	1
BP ± > 50% of normal	0
Consciousness	
Fully awake	2
Arousable on calling	1
Not responsive	0
Activity	
Moves all extremities	2
Moves two extremities	1
No movement	0

A total score of 9 or 10 shows readiness for discharge.

Table 3. Post-anesthetic Aldrete recovery score.

1.4. Special considerations for pediatric patients

When performing physical examinations on pediatric patients, it is critical to remember the differences between children at various ages and adults with regard to anatomy (e.g., airway), vital signs (e.g., heart and respiratory rates), and physiology (greater body surface area or mass and cardiac output). Cardiac output is more heart rate dependent in the child than in the adult. When assessing the child for anesthesia, the OMS must also pay particular attention to the patient's allergy history for the common childhood precipitants of asthmatic attacks: pollen, other indoor or outdoor airborne irritants, animal hair, physical exercise, and/or anxiety. Upper respiratory tract infections that produce airway irritability are exceedingly common in young children. Specific reactions to suspected drug allergens should be ascertained through allergy testing with, for example, an allergy panel. Noted differences between the pediatric and adult airways include: higher, more anterior position of the glottis opening in the child; relatively larger tongue in the infant; larger and more floppy epiglottis in the child; the subglottic region as the functionally narrowest portion of the pediatric airway versus the vocal cords in the adult; and larger relative size of the occiput in the infant.

1.5. Preoperative cardiac and pulmonary assessment

It comes as no surprise to the seasoned OMS/anesthesia provider that the two most important systems to consider on patient evaluation are the cardiac and pulmonary systems. Perioperative adverse cardiac events may occur in the OMFS patient. High-risk patients can usually be identified during a comprehensive history, review of systems, and physical examination. The history should elicit conditions such as stable (ASA 3) or unstable (ASA 4) angina, recent or past myocardial infarction with or without cardiac stent and appropriate anticoagulation, heart failure—compensated or decompensated, significant arrhythmias, valvular disease, and the presence of a pacemaker or a defibrillator. Patients should be questioned on their smoking status (current or former use, how many cigarettes per day, how many years), management and control of their blood sugars in diabetes mellitus, and renal insufficiency. Functional status should be quantified based on the metabolic equivalent (MET) (**Table 4**), which is used in the American College of Cardiology/American Heart Association Guidelines (ACC/AHA) [11]. For example, a person functioning at 1 MET is limited to simple activities such as eating, dressing, and using the toilet. A person with 4 METs can climb a flight of stairs, walk up a hill, or walk on level ground at 4 mph, and would generally not require an extensive cardiac workup. Physical examination should be used to look for jugular venous distention, arrhythmias, and abnormal heart sounds such as an S_3 gallop or murmur. The information obtained from the history and examination can be used to assess risk and to direct further testing.

MET	Functional levels of exercise
1	Eating, working at a computer, dressing
2	Walking down stairs or in your house, cooking
3	Walking 1–2 blocks
4	Raking leaves, gardening
5	Climbing 1 flight of stairs, dancing, bicycling
6	Playing golf, carrying clubs
7	Playing singles tennis

MET	Functional levels of exercise
8	Rapidly climbing stairs, jogging slowly
9	Jumping rope slowly, moderate cycling
10	Swimming quickly, running or jogging briskly
11	Skiing cross-country, playing full-court basketball
12	Running rapidly for moderate to long distances

MET, metabolic equivalent of the task. 1 MET is defined as the amount of oxygen consumed while sitting at rest and is equal to 3.5 mL O_2 per kilogram of body weight × min. The MET concept represents a simple, practical, and easily understood procedure for expressing the energy cost of physical activities as a multiple of the resting metabolic rate. The energy cost of an activity can be determined by dividing the relative oxygen cost of the activity (mL O_2/kg/min) by 3.5 [12].

Table 4. Estimated energy requirements for various activities (METs)

Indices for assessment of cardiac morbidity and mortality in noncardiac surgery have been established. The Revised Cardiac Risk Index (RCRI) is one such important assessment tool (**Table 5**). If it is determined that the patient is at significant risk for a postoperative cardiac event, further workup should be conducted and the condition should be optimized prior to the surgical procedure, if possible. Consultation with the patient's cardiologist should be sought when coronary or valvular disease is suspected or if assistance is needed with management of pacemakers or defibrillators.

Risk factors	
Ischemic heart disease	
Congestive heart failure	
Cerebrovascular disease	
Diabetes mellitus requiring preoperative insulin	
Serum creatinine > 2.0 mg/dL	
High-risk surgery (intraperitoneal, intrathoracic, or suprainguinal vascular)	
RCRI classification	**Event rate (%)**
Low risk (0 factors)	0.5
Low risk (1 factor)	1.3
Intermediate risk (2 factors)	3.6
High risk (3 or more factors)	9.1

Table 5. Revised Cardiac Risk Index (RCRI) [13].

1.6. Twelve-lead electrocardiogram (ECG)

A preoperative ECG is indicated within 30 days prior to the surgical procedure in patients with known coronary disease, peripheral vascular disease, or cerebrovascular disease. It may be reasonable to obtain an ECG in patients with a single clinical risk factor (e.g., diabetes mellitus, renal insufficiency, or congestive heart failure) who are to have an intermediate risk operation (more than "minor" oral surgical procedures). There is no evidence to support the routine use of ECG in patients without risk factors.

1.7. Noninvasive testing of left ventricular function

Evaluation of left ventricular function by radionuclide angiography or echocardiography is reasonable in patients with dyspnea of unknown origin or worsening dyspnea in the setting of known congestive heart failure (decompensated). The routine evaluation of left ventricular function is not otherwise indicated.

1.8. Noninvasive stress testing

Noninvasive stress testing involves radionuclide or echocardiographic imaging combined with pharmacologic stress to evaluate for ischemia and arrhythmias in patients who are unable to exercise. Patients with one or two clinical risk factors and poor functional capacity (<4 METs) should be considered for noninvasive stress testing. Routine noninvasive stress testing is not indicated in patients without clinical risk factors. Patients with active cardiac conditions should usually be evaluated by other methods.

1.9. Pulmonary and airway assessment

Patient-related risk factors for perioperative pulmonary complications include chronic obstructive pulmonary disease (COPD), pneumonia, sleep apnea, dyspnea, advanced age, obesity, and smoking [14, 15]. The most important part of a pulmonary risk assessment is a thorough history and physical examination. Specifically, the patient should be asked about shortness of breath, dyspnea on exertion, productive coughs, and symptoms of sleep apnea. A smoking history should also be obtained. Smoking cessation may reduce postoperative pulmonary complications. Patients experience increased mucociliary response and airway hypersensitivity shortly upon termination of smoking which will increase the risk of pulmonary complications. Ideally, patients should stop smoking for at least 8 weeks prior to the surgical procedure in order to reduce pulmonary morbidity.

Sleep apnea is a common and underdiagnosed problem [16]. Risk factors include obesity, male gender, a short/stout neck, macroglossia, and enlarged tonsils (**Table 6**). Symptoms and signs related to apnea are snoring, nighttime choking, or gasping, observed cessation of breathing by a partner, morning headaches, and daytime somnolence. Premedication with clonidine [17] given the night before and 2 h prior to surgery has been shown to reduce the need for operative anesthesia and to improve perioperative hemodynamics, anesthetic recovery, and pain control.

The Mallampati classification is a scoring system that relates the amount of mouth opening to the size of the tongue, and provides an estimate of space available for oral intubation by direct laryngoscopy. According to the Mallampati scale (**Figure 1**), class one is present when the soft palate, uvula, and pillars are visible, class two when the soft palate and base of the uvula are visible, class three when only the soft palate is visible, and class four when only the hard palate is visible.

Degree of tonsils blockage	Ratio of the tonsil in the oropharynx
Degree 0	Tonsils in the fossa
Degree 1	Tonsil occupies < 25% of the oropharynx
Degree 2	Tonsil occupies 25–50% of the oropharynx
Degree 3	Tonsil occupies 50–75% of the oropharynx
Degree 4	Tonsil occupies > 75% of the oropharynx

Table 6. Brodsky tonsil classification system

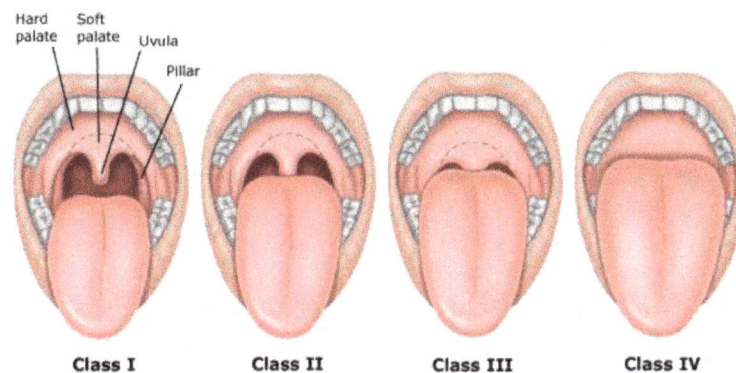

Figure 1. Mallampati classification.

1.10. Renal/endocrine systems assessment

Renal failure has been associated with increased risks of surgical infection and issues with wound healing [18]. It can also lead to disturbances in electrolytes and fluid balance, which may exacerbate the physiologic changes occurring during the perioperative period. In the patient with known or suspected renal failure, it may be prudent to evaluate the serum concentrations of the patient's potassium, magnesium, calcium, and phosphate. Blood urea nitrogen and creatinine assays should be obtained. Patients with newly diagnosed renal failure should be evaluated by a nephrologist prior to general anesthesia and surgery. Dialysis may be indicated if the uremia is found to be significant [19].

1.11. Diabetes and hyperglycemia

The prevalence of diabetes in the United States has been increasing and is currently estimated to be about 10%. Many more individuals likely remain undiagnosed. Hyperglycemia has been associated with immune dysfunction, elevation of inflammatory markers, vascular endothelium dysfunction, and thrombosis. Clinically, hyperglycemia can lead to increased surgical site infection and postoperative mortality [20–23].

At-risk patients should be assessed for hyperglycemia prior to surgery. Known diabetics should have their hemoglobin A1c levels evaluated along with a fasting serum glucose test. Optimization of blood glucose control prior to surgical intervention should be undertaken, if possible. For nondiabetic patients at risk of hyperglycemia (e.g., the obese and the elderly), consideration should be given to measuring the preoperative and intraoperative fasting glucose level. If these levels are found to be elevated, measures to tightly control serum glucose (e.g., insulin infusion) should be initiated [21, 22, 24].

1.12. Summary of preoperative assessment

Risk evaluation should be done for every OMFS patient. A diligent evaluation using the presented guidelines will allow optimization of care throughout the perioperative period. The ultimate goal of achieving improved outcomes should encourage the consistent assessment of all potential risk factors for each patient.

2. Sedation

2.1. Levels of sedation

The American Dental Association (ADA) has incorporated the American Society of Anesthesiology (ASA) definitions for use in its own published guidelines. The categorization as detailed by both the ASA and ADA focuses on the concept that the spectrum of sedation and anesthesia is a continuum extending from mild sedation (anxiolysis) to moderate sedation and analgesia ("conscious sedation") to deep sedation and analgesia to general anesthesia. The ASA and ADA differentiate these levels based on four parameters, which measure responsiveness, airway integrity, spontaneous ventilation, and cardiovascular hemodynamics (**Table 7**).

Minimal sedation (anxiolysis) is a drug-induced state during which patients respond normally to verbal commands. Although cognitive function and physical coordination may be impaired, airway reflexes, ventilatory, and cardiovascular functions are unaffected.

Moderate sedation/analgesia ("conscious sedation") is a drug-induced depression of consciousness during which patients respond purposefully to verbal commands, either alone or accompanied by light tactile stimulation. No interventions are required to maintain a patent airway, and spontaneous ventilation is adequate. Cardiovascular function is usually maintained.

Deep sedation/analgesia is a drug-induced depression of consciousness during which patients cannot be easily aroused but respond purposefully following repeated or painful stimulation. The ability to independently maintain ventilatory function may be impaired. Patients may require assistance in maintaining a patent airway, and spontaneous ventilation may be inadequate. Cardiovascular function is usually maintained.

General anesthesia is a drug-induced loss of consciousness during which patients are not arousable, even by painful stimulation. The ability to independently maintain ventilatory function is often impaired. Patients often require assistance in maintaining a patent airway, and positive pressure ventilation may be required because of depressed spontaneous ventilation or drug-induced depression of neuromuscular function. Cardiovascular function may be impaired.

Characteristic	Minimal sedation	Moderate sedation and analgesia	Deep sedation and analgesia	General anesthesia
Responsiveness	Normal response to verbal stimulation	Purposeful response to verbal or tactile stimulation	Purposeful response after repeated or painful stimulation	Unarousable even with painful stimulus
Airway	Unaffected	No intervention required	Intervention may be required	Intervention often required
Spontaneous ventilation	Unaffected	Adequate	May be inadequate	Frequently inadequate
Cardiovascular function	Unaffected	Usually maintained	Usually maintained	May be impaired

Reproduced with permission of *Anesthesiology* from the American Society of Anesthesiologists Task Force on Sedation and Analgesia by Non-anesthesiologists

†Reflex withdrawal from a painful stimulus is not considered a purposeful response

Table 7. Continuum of depth of sedation: definition of general anesthesia and levels of sedation and analgesia

In most situations, the primary goal of outpatient sedation in the OMFS office is to achieve comfort and cooperation which is accomplished by a drug-induced alteration in consciousness. Responsiveness can be used as the primary parameter to assess the state of consciousness, which defines the desired anesthetic level. The terms mild, moderate, deep, and general descriptively imply both the desired response and depth of sedation. Given sufficient anesthetic medications, a patient will proceed from a state of relaxation with a normal response to verbal stimulation to a state in which they are unarousable.

Most anesthetic agents cause airway musculature relaxation and depress the hypoxic and hypercapnic respiratory drive, which have the potential to impair airway integrity and patency as well as spontaneous ventilation. As the level of sedation becomes deeper, both airway patency and spontaneous ventilation may and will ultimately require intervention and assistance.

Sedation is a continuous spectrum, and there is always a danger for the patient's airway to become compromised, which can go unnoticed in the absence of diligent monitoring. In addition, patient responsiveness and depth of anesthesia fluctuate depending on the level of stimulation. When the patient is more responsive, there may be a temptation to administer additional sedative medication. However, sustained procedural stimulation is rare and if additional anesthetic medication is administered to diminish patient responsiveness, respiratory depression may result upon cessation of the procedural stimulation. This presents one of the limitations with the lighter levels of sedation as patient comfort and cooperation may be unachievable without infringing on the potential of adverse events.

It is important for the OMS to be cognizant that levels of sedation are independent of the route of administration or the selection of anesthetic agent. The OMS must also be cognizant that there is a wide variability in patient response to the various anesthetic medications, which could produce a more profoundly sedated patient than desired or anticipated.

2.2. Monitoring in OMFS sedation

The OMS/anesthesia provider is responsible for continuously monitoring the sedated patient. This consists of direct observation as well as utilization and interpretation of cardiovascular and respiratory monitors. Adverse respiratory events have been the primary etiology resulting in adverse outcomes. Standard of care in OMFS offices dictates that the following monitors be applied: pulse oximeter, noninvasive blood pressure monitoring, electrocardiography, capnography, and pretracheal stethoscope auscultation.

Pulse oximetry has been the standard of care for monitoring oxygen saturation for almost three decades. Pulse oximetry measures the amount of oxygen carried by hemoglobin molecules in arterial blood (oxygen saturation), which is displayed as a percentage. Arterial oxygen content is inferred (but not directly measured) from the percent hemoglobin saturation on the oxygen-hemoglobin dissociation curve.

Partial or complete airway obstruction and ventilatory depression from anesthetic medication, if not remediated, will result in an eventual decrease in arterial oxygen content which can be detected by pulse oximetry. However, it is important to realize that there will be at least a 20–30-s delay in the detection of these events as pulse oximetry measures hemoglobin saturation at the fingertip where blood may take up to 20–30 s to travel from the core circulation. Administration of supplemental oxygen will further postpone the onset of desaturation with airway obstruction or ventilatory compromise. For these reasons, pulse oximetry is not an efficient ventilatory monitor.

Ventilation is the movement of gas in and out of the lungs. Ventilatory monitoring for deep sedation and general anesthesia can be best accomplished with both capnography and a pretracheal stethoscope. Capnography typically utilizes infrared gas analysis technology to assess the concentration of carbon dioxide in inspired and expired air. The capnographic unit provides both an absolute end-tidal carbon dioxide ($ETCO_2$) value as well as a graphic demonstration of the patient's ventilation pattern (**Table 8**). In an open system (e.g., nonintubated patient), the exhaled air may be diluted with ambient air, minimizing the benefit of capnography; however, the graphic display can provide visual cues for the respiratory rate as well as an impairment of gas exchange (e.g., obstruction, bronchospasm). In addition, changes in ventilation, such as a change in the graphic display suggestive of airway obstruction, are detected and displayed immediately. The practitioner must be cognizant that capnography can fail in an open system as there is no direct sealed conduit between alveoli and the monitor.

The combination of both capnography and pretracheal auscultation improves the accuracy of ventilatory monitoring, as $ETCO_2$ sampled from the nose in a mouth breather can be inaccurate, and pretracheal auscultation during slow ventilation in an open airway can be silent or difficult to hear.

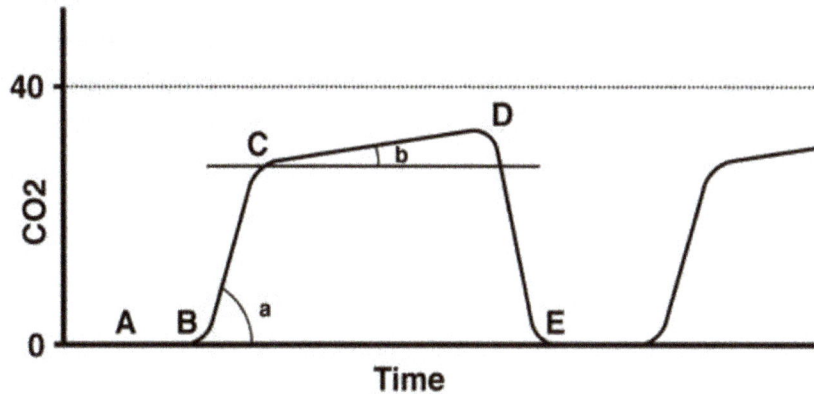

Table 8. End tidal CO_2 monitor graphical recording

3. Anesthetic agents

3.1. Clinical summary

An administered drug's activity is determined by its ability to cross the blood-brain barrier (degree of lipid solubility) to reach and bind respective central nervous system (CNS) receptors [the "vessel rich" group receives 75% of cardiac output (CO)] in sufficient concentration to exert its intended actions such as analgesia, sedation, hypnosis, and/or amnesia. A drug's side effects are usually due to its action at locations other than its targeted receptors. A drug's action is also dependent on the dose given, the rate of administration, and receptor number and

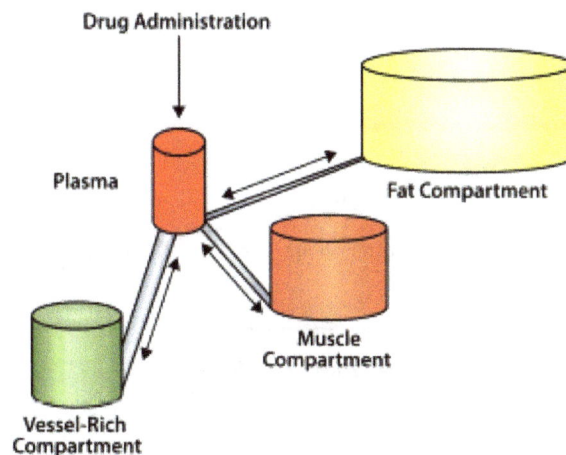

Figure 2. Drug distribution to various body compartments.

sensitivity, with a wide range of variability among patients. The actions of most short-acting drugs are terminated by redistribution ($T_{1/2}\alpha$) to other compartments (**Figure 2**). Longer-acting drugs are terminated by metabolism ($T_{1/2}\beta$) in the liver into smaller, water soluble moieties which can then be filtered and excreted by the kidney (or in sweat, mucus from the lungs, and gastrointestinal excretions to a small extent). Drugs may also "hide" in muscular (20% of CO), adipose (5% of CO) tissues or remain bound to plasma proteins (**Figure 3**), in which cases the intended receptors are not activated and clinical effects are absent (**Figure 4**). "Hidden drugs" can subsequently redistribute from "hidden reservoirs" prior to metabolism, causing a return or additive clinical effect also known as hangover. Hypoproteinemia (e.g., cachexia, anorexia, liver disease) will similarly enhance drug availability and action.

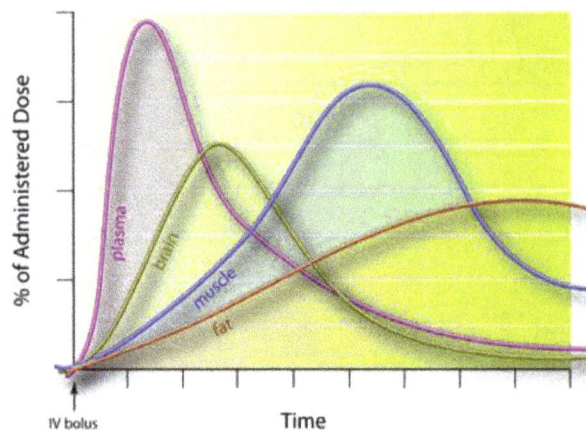

Figure 3. Drug distribution to various compartments over time.

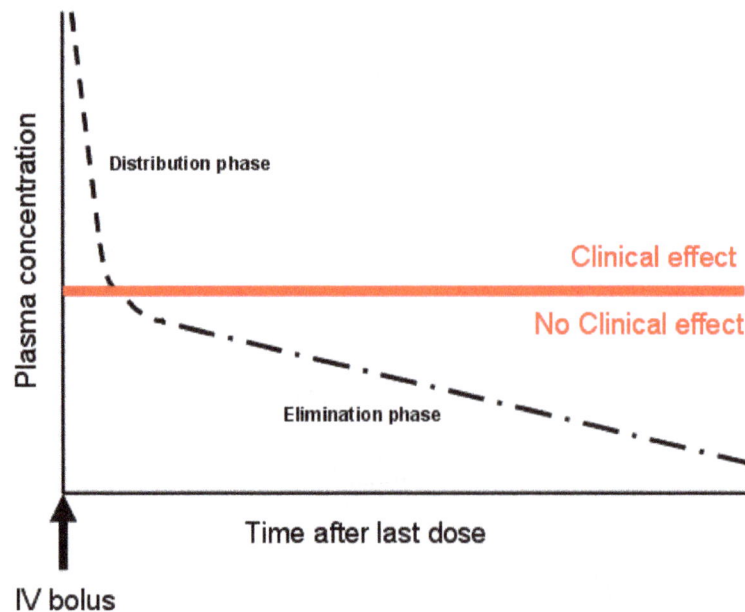

Figure 4. Plasma drug concentration versus time after an intravenous (IV) dose.

4. Review of anesthetic medications

This section focuses on describing many of the characteristics and properties of some of the most commonly used in-OMFS-office sedatives. The list of medications described here is not intended to be exclusive. The authors realize that with variations in OMFS training programs, variations in preferred drug regimens exist.

4.1. Benzodiazepines

Mechanism of action: bind to and enhance $GABA_A$ receptors to the actions of GABA ("GABAergic"), increase chloride conductance, and hyperpolarize neurons, thereby interrupting nerve transmissions. Benzodiazepines can be described as agonists of inhibitory GABA receptors.

Intended effects include sedation, anxiolysis, anterograde amnesia, muscle relaxation, and anticonvulsant activity. Benzodiazepines exert minimal cardiovascular effects and respiratory depression (decreased tidal volume and increased respiratory rate). They suppress psychotomimetic ketamine effects.

Adverse side effects include minimal cardiovascular or respiratory changes when used alone in therapeutic dose; however, benzodiazepines are synergistic with other agents. A paradoxical excitement (disinhibition) reaction is possible in patients at age extremes and in anxious teenage patients.

Benzodiazepines are metabolized via the liver and are excreted renally.

Midazolam: Water soluble until aromatic ring closes at pH > 4 (after injection), which enhances lipid solubility. Can be given by mouth (PO), intravenously (IV), or intramuscularly (IM). Midazolam has minimally active metabolites. Adult sedation/anxiolysis: 5 mg or 0.07 mg/kg IM; or 1 mg IV slowly q2–3 min up to 5 mg. Pediatric premedication dose ~0.25–1.0 mg/kg up to 20 mg maximum PO, or 0.1–0.15 mg/kg IM. Midazolam has an IV onset time of 1.5–5 min, peak effects at 4–8 min, and duration of 15–20 min.

Diazepam: Diazepam is a lipid soluble agent that requires propylene glycol to dissolve in water, which in turn creates a risk for thrombophlebitis. It features erratic IM absorption but can be given PO, IV, or IM. Physiologically, diazepam is metabolized to oxydiazepam, which is an active metabolite and contributes to a longer duration of action and hangover compared to midazolam. Diazepam has an IV onset time of 1.5–5 min, peak effects at 3–5 min, and duration of 15–60 min.

4.2. Flumazenil

Flumazenil is an inhibitory agonist of the GABA-benzodiazepine receptor complex (specifically) with no intrinsic activity. It will occupy a "free" receptor but will not displace other agonists and is therefore not very effective for quick reversal after an overdose. It is characterized by its high affinity, short duration, and possible contraindication in patients with seizure disorders as it may trigger seizures in patients who rely on benzodiazepines for seizure control. Other side effects may include agitation, arrhythmias, and dizziness, pain on injection, nausea/vomiting (N/V), sweating, headaches, and blurred vision. The dose for benzodiazepine sedation reversal is 0.2 mg IV over 15 s, then 0.2 mg q1 min as needed up to 1 mg total dose. The dose for benzodiazepine overdose reversal is 0.2 mg IV over 30 s, then 0.3–0.5 mg q30 s as needed up to 3 mg total dose.

4.3. Opioids

Mechanism of action: opioid medications bind to multiple opioid receptors, most notably at the central nervous system (brain and spinal cord) mu receptors.

Intended effects of opioids include analgesia, attenuation of the neuroendocrine stress response, blunted laryngeal reflex, sedation, euphoria, and mental clouding. Opioids also provide cardiovascular stability.

Adverse side effects include vagal nerve mediated bradycardia, decreased sympathetic tone (decrease in systemic vascular resistance leading to hypotension), pupillary constriction, respiratory depression (blunted response to hypercarbia), N/V, muscular rigidity with rapid or high dosing (which initiates at the small muscles of the larynx then progresses to the chest wall and skeletal muscles), pruritus, histamine release (seen with morphine and meperidine).

The majority of opioids are metabolized via the liver, though remifentanil is metabolized in the plasma.

4.4. Opioid receptors include the following: mu, delta, kappa, sigma

Mu (μ) receptors are located primarily in the brainstem and medial thalamus. Binding to these lead to supraspinal analgesia, respiratory depression, euphoria, sedation, decreased gastro-intestinal motility, and physical dependence.

Delta (δ) receptors are localized largely in the basal ganglia and the neocortical regions of the brain, though their effects are not well studied. It is believed they may be responsible for psychomimetic and dysphoric effects.

Kappa (k) receptors are located in the limbic and other diencephalic areas, the brain stem, and the spinal cord. They primarily induce spinal analgesia, sedation, dyspnea, dependence, dysphoria, and respiratory depression.

Sigma (Σ) receptors have been described as being responsible for dysphoria and hypertonia.

Fentanyl is a commonly used in-office synthetic opioid medication (phenylpiperidine class) that is 100 times more potent than morphine (phenanthrene class). It acts at a variety of receptors within the central nervous system (mu, kappa, delta, and sigma). It produces venodilation, a decrease in heart rate via vagal response, and respiratory depression (dose dependent). It affects respiratory rate more than tidal volume, decreases stress response to surgery, and is metabolized by the liver to be excreted in the urine and bile. Potential side effects include: cough-suppression, constipation, urinary retention, biliary tract spasm, and muscle rigidity. It has an IV onset time of 5+ min, peak effects at 6 min, and duration of approximately 1 h.

Remifentanil is an atypical phenylpiperidine opioid that is metabolized by plasma esterases. It must be delivered as an IV bolus or via continuous infusion. Apnea and hypotension are more common with remifentanil than with other opioids. It has a very rapid onset (due to a small volume of distribution that is 1/10 that of fentanyl) and offset (esterase metabolism) and has a clearance that is more than 2.5 times as rapid as the other opioids'. It has an IV onset time of 1 min, offset time of 5+ min, peak effects at <1 min, and duration of 3–5 min regardless of the duration of infusion, age, or renal and hepatic status. It is supplied as a powder that must be reconstituted.

Meperidine is a pure synthetic opioid that has an active metabolite, normeperidine, which has half the potency but possesses proconvulsant potential. Meperidine has a slight anticholinergic effect, releases histamine, slightly elevates heart rate, and can be effective for controlling postoperative/post-anesthetic shivering, xerostomia, and mydriasis. It is contraindicated for us with monoamine oxidase inhibitors (MAOIs) as both drugs will increase serotonin and can trigger serotonin syndrome (too much serotonin), which consists of cognitive (confusion, agitation, and lethargy), autonomic (hyperadrenergic state), and somatic (myoclonic, twitching, and tremor) symptoms. It has an IV onset time of 5 min and duration of 2–3 h.

4.5. Opioid antagonist

Naloxone is a competitive antagonist of all opioid receptors—it can displace an agonist if the affinity and/or concentration of this antagonist are greater than the affinity and/or concentration of the agonist. The resultant effect is the reversal of the analgesic and ventilatory depressant effects of the opioid. There is a concern about a possible premature termination of the antagonistic effects. If naloxone is used to rescue overdose-induced ventilatory insufficiency, the practitioner must monitor the patient for an additional 1–2 h to ensure against re-sedation. Possible side effects can include flash pulmonary edema (usually in patients with cardiovascular diseases), dysphoria and withdrawal symptoms (in patients who are dependent on opioids for chronic pain relief and where rapid reversal will trigger intense pain), and sympathetic hypertension with possible pulmonary consequences. The usual dosing for adult post-op reversal is 0.1–0.2 mg q2–3 min as needed. Its duration is 30–45 min.

4.6. NMDA receptor antagonist

Ketamine is a phencyclidine derivative. Its pharmacodynamics involves analgesia, anesthesia, and sympathomimetic effects that are mediated by different receptor sites. Non-competitive NMDA (N-methyl-D-aspartate) receptor antagonism is associated with the analgesic effects, opiate receptors may contribute to analgesia and dysphoric reactions, and sympathomimetic properties may result from enhanced central and peripheral monoaminergic transmission. Ketamine blocks dopamine reuptake and therefore elevates synaptic dopamine levels [25]. Inhibition of central and peripheral cholinergic transmission could contribute to induction of the anesthetic state and hallucinations [26]. Ketamine is structurally similar to PCP (phencyclidine), but 10–50 times less potent in blocking NMDA effects. The exact mechanism of action is unclear. Ketamine produces dissociative anesthesia between the thalamocortical and limbic systems; that is, patients do not perceive painful, visual, or auditory stimuli and appear to be in a cataleptic state. Ketamine is also a direct myocardial depressant. Central sympathomimetics cause a non-dose dependent increase in the heart rate, cardiac output, and blood pressure. It relaxes bronchial smooth muscles but has a minimal effect on the respiratory drive. Ketamine's expected effects are excellent analgesia [27], strong anterograde amnesia, preserved laryngeal reflexes, suppression of convulsive neuronal activities, increased intraocular and intracranial pressures, and increased salivation and lacrimation. Its adverse effects include possible emergence delirium (especially seen with large doses in elderly and pediatric patients, females, and those with underlying personality disorders [28]), dose-related increases in muscle tone, random non-triggered movements, nausea, and vomiting. For common in-office OMFS sedation use, usual dosage (the "low dose IV regimen") is 0.1–0.5 mg/kg which is most often combined with additional benzodiazepines, an opioid, and propofol. Dosages of 1–2 mg/kg IV over 1–2 min or 4 mg/kg IM induce 10–20 min of a dissociative state. Its onset time is very rapid (<1 min), and its duration is 10–15 min. Ketamine is metabolized in the liver and is renally excreted.

4.7. Imidazole derivatives

Etomidate is a GABA agonist that is used for rapid induction of dose-dependent sedation/anesthesia when hypotension cannot be tolerated and cardiovascular stability must be maintained after bolus induction. It has a wide therapeutic index and is the induction agent of choice in patients with severe cardiovascular disease. Induction IV dose is 0.3 mg/kg with maintenance dosing of 5–20 μg/kg/min. It is metabolized by the liver and in plasma and is renally excreted. Possible adrenocortical suppression can be observed, especially when combined with benzodiazepines and opioids. Other potential side effects and precautions include injection pain and phlebitis, hiccups, myoclonic activity on induction, nausea, and vomiting.

4.8. Barbiturates

Barbiturates are both GABAergic and GABAmimetic—they do not require GABA for their intended effects. They are very lipophilic, producing rapid on and offsets but will accumulate in adipose tissue and can lead to a prolonged hangover with high doses.

Intended effects of barbiturates include hypnosis and anticonvulsant properties with no histamine release.

Possible adverse side effects include hyperalgesia in subanesthetic doses (paradoxical excitement), pain on injection (alkaline pH of 11), hypotension (especially with hypovolemia) with compensatory tachycardia, dose-dependent respiratory depression, and excitatory phenomenon such as tremors, twitching, heightened airway reflexes, and laryngospasm.

Methohexital is an ultra-short acting barbiturate that acts by GABA receptor activation and increasing chloride ion channels. It has a rapid onset (1 min) and offset (5–8 min) but does not accumulate in adipose tissue. Expected effects include venodilation, increases in heart rate with stable cardiac output, and central depression of respiratory rate and tidal volume. Methohexital is safe for asthmatics (no histamine release) but does not produce bronchodilation. It is contraindicated in patients with acute intermittent porphyria. Adverse side effects may include nausea/vomiting, laryngospasm, bronchospasm, hiccups, and apnea. It is metabolized by the liver.

4.9. Sedative

Propofol (2, 6 diisopropylphenol) is a short acting ($T_{1/2}\alpha$ 2–8 min, $T_{1/2}\beta$ 4–7 h) hypnotic general anesthetic agent that increases the function of GABA receptors. It is GABAergic and GABA-mimetic and may inhibit the NMDA receptor. It does not provide analgesia or antalgesia but does produce sedation, amnesia, hypnosis, and is a profound antiemetic. There is notable dose-dependent respiratory depression, and it may produce apnea on induction. Propofol also helps relax bronchial smooth muscle and is safe to use with asthmatics (no histamine release). Systolic blood pressure may be reduced 20–40% by blocked sympathetic tone (hypotension without compensatory tachycardia); this effect may be more exaggerated in the medically compromised and elderly patients. Propofol may also reduce the heart rate by 20%. There is a more rapid awakening with propofol and less residual central nervous system side effects with only mild euphoria. There is a low incidence of N/V but patients may experience pain on injection if given in large bolus doses. Propofol is manufactured with no anti-microbial preservatives; therefore, it must be discarded after 6 h once drawn up. As some formulations contain soy or egg products, it may be prudent to use great caution in exposing allergic patients to such solutions. IV sedation infusion dose: 5–50 mcg/kg/min; deep sedation bolus dose: 1 mg/kg IV over 20–30 s, repeat 0.5 mg/kg IV as needed.

4.10. Succinylcholine

Succinylcholine is comprised of two acetylcholine molecules joined together and acts as a depolarizing neuromuscular blocker by binding acetylcholine receptors at the post-synaptic neuromuscular junction end plate. The resultant end plate depolarization initially stimulates muscle contraction; however, because succinylcholine is not degraded by acetylcholinesterase, it remains in the neuromuscular junction to maintain continuous end plate depolarization and subsequent muscle relaxation referred to as a "Phase I Block." Succinylcholine is metabolized by pseudocholinesterase. Its effects may be prolonged in approximately 20% of patients because of atypical or deficient expression of the pseudocholinesterase enzyme. This defect may be diagnosed via the use of the local anesthetic dibucaine, which drastically reduces the action of normal plasma cholinesterase. An atypical patient will not experience the full effects of dibucaine.

Succinylcholine use is a potential etiology behind hyperkalemia and cardiac arrest with expected 0.5–1 mEq/L increases in serum potassium levels following administration. This effect may be exaggerated in patients with neuropathies, denervation injuries, dystrophies, myopathies, strabismus, end-stage renal disease, and burns over a week old as a result of increased acetylcholine receptor expression.

4.11. Volatile anesthetic (VA) agents

With the exception of nitrous oxide (N_2O), inhaled anesthetics do not provide any significant analgesia, though they produce immobility and amnesia. Other than N_2O (which increases skeletal muscle tone), inhaled anesthetics do not affect or, in some cases, decrease skeletal muscle tone. Volatile anesthetic (VA) agents produce immobility via actions on the spinal cord and anesthesia by enhancing inhibitory channels and attenuating excitatory channels. Whether or not this occurs through direct binding or membrane alterations is not known. VAs also depress the cardiovascular system, thereby reducing the mean arterial pressure. Desflurane, isoflurane, and sevoflurane decrease the systemic vascular resistance, which is reflected by a decrease in blood pressure. VAs cause dose-dependent decreases in ventilation. They lead to decreases in tidal volume and compensatory increases in respiratory rate, but a net decrease in min ventilation. A decrease in minute ventilation causes an increase in CO_2.

Ventilation is the most important factor affecting the elimination and dilution of sevoflurane, desflurane, and isoflurane. The time needed for a 50% decrease in sevoflurane, desflurane, or isoflurane is <5 min and essentially independent of case duration. The rate of onset of VAs is indirectly proportional to the blood/gas partition coefficient as a lower coefficient corresponds to rapid equilibration between alveolar gas and capillary blood. The rate is directly proportional to the oil/water partition coefficient as a higher oil/water partition signifies a more rapid uptake through the BBB. All three agents are bronchodilators in general anesthetic doses. However, desflurane and isoflurane are pungent and, upon induction, may precipitate bronchospasm and/or laryngospasm. VAs carry the very serious risk of developing malignant hyperthermia (MH). This risk is decreased with desflurane and sevoflurane (and possibly isoflurane) as compared to halothane, though all potent volatile agents should be avoided in the MH-susceptible patient.

Agent	MAC (potency)	Blood-gas partition coefficient (solubility)
Nitrogen	–	0.014 (least soluble)
Desflurane	6.0	0.42
Nitrous oxide	105 (least potent)	0.47
Sevoflurane	2.0	0.65
Isoflurane	1.2	1.4 (most soluble)

MAC: minimum alveolar concentration.

Table 9. Comparison of various common anesthetic agents, potency, and solubility

In general, volatile agents can exist in two phases: gaseous and in solution. The proportion of the agent in its gas phase compared to those dissolved in blood is determined by the blood/gas partition coefficient, which is described using solubility and ambient pressure. If an agent is largely soluble, it resides in solution and exerts no measurable pressure. Pressure—gas tension in an enclosed space—is necessary to drive movement of agents across membranes.

Highly soluble agents are slower in onset and offset, but conversely, they may be held more extensively within the circulating blood. **Table 9** compares various anesthetic gases, their potency, and their solubility.

4.12. MAC

The potency of anesthetic gases are often described using the minimum alveolar concentration (MAC), defined as the concentration of an anesthetic gas administered at 1 atmosphere of ambient pressure required to prevent skeletal muscle movement in response to pain (e.g., surgical skin incision) in 50% of patients. Factors that can increase the MAC include fever, young age, hyperadrenergic states, and chronic alcohol abuse while anemia, old age, hypotension, and other anesthetic agents (such as narcotics, propofol) can lead to its decrease.

4.13. Second gas effect into nitrogen-filled spaces

Nitrogen (N_2) is the least soluble gas and therefore diffuses most rapidly. Nitrous oxide (N_2O) also diffuses rapidly relative to halogenated vapors as the next least soluble gas. When N_2O leaves the alveoli more rapidly than other gases can enter, it creates a gaseous void that shrinks the alveolar volume and increases the concentration (partial pressure) of other gases present, subsequently facilitating their diffusion down the newly amplified concentration gradients. This contributes to the movement of slower moving, more soluble agents, which also creates/enhances a void that theoretically can cause a follow-up "Venturi effect" on other gases. Although N_2 moves more quickly than N_2O because it is less soluble, N_2O is carried in greater concentration in blood; hence, the rate determining step of N_2O moving in more quickly than N_2 moving out is in the blood flow and has little to do with relative solubility differences. N_2O moving in more quickly than N_2 moving out expands compliant nitrogen-filled spaces and pressurizes non-complaint nitrogen-filled spaces.

Nitrous oxide (N_2O) is a GABAergic anesthetic agent that is an NMDA antagonist. It provides analgesia and anxiolysis but can be emetogenic in higher doses. It works in synergy with other volatile anesthetic agents via the second gas effect to lower the MAC. No increased cardiovascular risk has been shown to result from its use; however, increased pressure is noted in non-compliant spaces such as the eyes, middle ears (especially with obstructed Eustachian tubes), and non-draining sinuses. Also noted is increased volume in compliant spaces such as air emboli, pulmonary blebs, bowel distension, and tamponading gas bubbles following retinal surgery. When used in higher elevations/altitudes, the concentration of N_2O must be higher because of less atmospheric pressure needed to drive gas diffusion.

4.14. Anticholinergics

Glycopyrrolate is a quaternary ammonium compound that does not cross the blood-brain barrier (BBB) and causes no sedation. Glycopyrrolate has a delayed onset and possesses more anti-sialagogue effect (its main indication for OMFS in-office use) and less tachycardia than atropine does. Expected effects with glycopyrrolate include tachycardia, bronchodilation, and a reduction in salivary flow. It is metabolized in the liver and renally excreted. Potential side effects include blurred vision, urinary retention, xerostomia, xerophthalmia, and tachycardia. Dosing for routine use as an anti-sialagogue is 0.1–0.2 mg (0.5–1.0 mL) IV.

Atropine is a tertiary ammonium compound that crosses the BBB. It has a rapid onset but possesses less anti-sialagogue effect and more tachycardia than glycopyrrolate. Expected effects with atropine include tachycardia, bronchodilation, and a smaller reduction in salivary flow. It is metabolized in the liver and renally excreted. Potential side effects include sedation/dysphoria, blurred vision, urinary retention, xerostomia, xerophthalmia, and hyper-vagal responses (tachycardia) with very small doses. Dosing for routine use as an anti-sialagogue is 0.4 mg via IV (1 mL).

4.15. Gastric prokinetics

Metoclopramide is a moderate central dopamine receptor (D_2) antagonist. It increases lower esophageal sphincter tone and upper gastrointestinal forward peristalsis. It is metabolized by the liver and is renally excreted. It must be avoided in patients with Parkinson's disease, and it may cause extrapyramidal reactions. Usual adult dose is 10 mg IV/IM.

4.16. Antiemetics

Patients at increased risk of perioperative/perianesthetic N/V include children, women, the obese, expectant mothers, gastroesophageal reflux disease (GERD) patients, those with a history of motion sickness, gastroparesis, the anxious, and those in acute pain.

Causes of perioperative/perianesthetic N/V include early ambulation, acute pain, unpleasant visual sights, odors, tastes, and physical stimulation of the pharynx. Anesthesia-related causes of N/V include high concentrations of N_2O, opioids, ketamine, gastric insufflation, hypoxia, and hypovolemia. Various surgical stimuli can also account for perioperative N/V. These might include blood in stomach (could be common following oral surgical procedures), throat drape that applies too much pressure on the skin over the larynx, and a Weider tongue retractor placed too deeply or too aggressively.

Treatment of perioperative N/V focuses on the following goals: prevent aspiration, avoid protracted recovery, prevent hypoxia, prevent hypovolemia, achieve meticulous hemostasis, prevent distress to patient, and correction of any possible electrolyte imbalances.

Ondansetron is a serotonin 5-HT3 receptor antagonist used to prevent N/V. It is produced in various forms, both for IV (4 mg) use as well as in oral dissolving tablets (8 mg). It is metabolized in the liver and renally excreted. It has no significant drug interactions and only demonstrates mild side effects such as constipation, dizziness, and headache.

Promethazine is a neuroleptic medication and a first generation histamine H_1 receptor antagonist. It has antiemetic and anticholinergic properties via actions on the Dopamine D_2 receptor. Promethazine can have an additive central nervous system action when combined with antidepressant medications. It is metabolized in the liver and is renally excreted. Possible side effects include excessive sedation, xerostomia, constipation, and rare neuroleptic malignant syndrome. It is recommended to avoid IV push when administering this medication as extravasation can lead to tissue necrosis. For parenteral use, the IM route in encouraged. Usual dosage is 6.25–25 mg IV, and 12.5–50 mg PO/IM/PR.

Diphenhydramine is a first generation antihistamine and an H_1 receptor antagonist. Antagonism is achieved through inhibiting the effects of histamine more so than its production or release. Diphenhydramine inhibits most smooth muscle vasoconstrictor effects of histamine. This antagonism may also produce anticholinergic effects, antiemetic effects, and significant sedative side effects [29, 30]. Diphenhydramine is metabolized in the liver and renally excreted. Usual adult dosage is 6.25–25 mg IV, and 12.5–50 mg PO/IM/PR.

Dexamethasone is a glucocorticoid and a well-established antiemetic in patients receiving highly emetogenic cancer chemotherapy. Its antiemetic mechanism of action is not well understood. Dexamethasone may antagonize prostaglandin, stimulate the release endorphins that improve mood and a sense of well-being, and stimulate appetite. It is metabolized in the liver and is renally excreted. It may incur interactions with non-steroidal anti-inflammatory medications, and potential side effects include hyperglycemia and euphoria/mania. Usual adult dose is 2–10 mg IM/IV, and 4–10 mg PO.

4.17. Local anesthetics

Local anesthetics (LA) are classified as either esters or amides. Esters include Novocain, procaine, benzocaine, and tetracaine. They are metabolized by plasma pseudocholinesterase. Amides include lidocaine, mepivacaine, and bupivacaine. They are metabolized in the liver by its microsomal enzymes. A commonly used LA, articaine, contains both an amide and an ester link but is classified as an amide.

The mechanism of action of LAs is that once they are injected into tissue, they exist in both ionized and nonionized forms. The nonionized base is able to penetrate many layers of tissue —the lipid nerve sheath and membrane. Re-equilibration between the ionized and nonionized forms occurs once passage is completed. While in the nerve axon, the ionized form is able to block sodium channels, prevent the inflow of sodium, slow the rate of depolarization, and thus preventing an action potential from occurring.

Agent	Lipid solubility	Protein binding	Duration	pKa	Onset time
Mepivacaine	1	75	Medium	7.6	Fast
Lidocaine	4	65	Medium	7.7	Fast
Bupivacaine	28	95	Long	8.1	Moderate

Table 10. Properties of local anesthetics

An ideal LA is one that is very potent, has a quick onset time, and has an appropriate duration of action sufficient to accomplish the procedural goals and then wear off with no permanent adverse effects. Properties often used to compare one LA to another include potency, duration, and onset time (**Table 10**). Potency is determined by lipid solubility. Greater lipid solubility produces a more potent LA (bupivacaine > lidocaine > mepivacaine). Duration is determined by the protein binding. Greater protein binding creates a longer duration (bupivacaine > mepivacaine > lidocaine). Onset time is determined by pKa. The closer the pKa of a LA is to the pH of tissue (7.4), the more rapid the onset (mepivacaine > lidocaine > bupivacaine). The pKa is the pH at which equal concentrations of ionized and nonionized forms exist.

Anesthetic	pKa	% Conc	Vasoconst	Pulpal (P)/Soft Tissue (ST) duration (min)	Max dose (mg/kg)	Max dose (absolute, mg)
Articaine	7.8	4	Epi 1:100k	P: 60–75 ST: 180–360	7 (adult)	500 (adult)
Bupivacaine	8.1	0.5	Epi 1:200k	P: 90–180 ST: 240–540	1.3 (adult)	90 (adult)
Lidocaine	7.7	2	None	P: 5–10, ST:60–120	4.5 (adult)	300 (adult)
		2	Epi 1:100k	P: 60, ST: 180–300	7.0 (adult)	500 (adult)
Mepivacaine	7.6	2	Levo 1:20k	P: 60, ST: 180–300	6.6	400
		3	None	P: 20–40, ST: 120–180	6.6	400
Prilocaine	7.9	4	None	P: 10–15 (infil), 40–60 (block); ST: 90–120 (infil), 120–240 (block)	6.0	400

Table 11. Comparison of various commonly used local anesthetics

Time	Blood levels of LA	Signs/symptoms
Initial	Minimal to moderate overdose	↑ HR, ↑ BP, ↑ RR Drowsiness, confusion, slurred speech, stuttering, talkative, excited, nystagmus, tinnitus, metallic taste
Progressive	Moderate overdose	Tremors, hallucinations, ↓ BP, ↓ HR, ↓ CO
Late	Moderate to high overdose	Unconsciousness, seizures, ventricular dysrhythmias, respiratory and circulatory arrest

Table 12. Clinical manifestations of local anesthetic toxicity

The most common drugs utilized by OMSs are LAs, so a detailed and intimate knowledge of these agents is essential to ensure a successful practice (**Table 11**). Occasionally, providers do not take into account special patient factors such as age, weight, or medical comorbidities; LA toxicity may result if maximum dosages are exceeded. Clinical manifestations of systemic LA toxicity are varied and may include only the (early) classic sign of circumoral numbness.

However, if left unnoticed, toxicity symptoms may progress and can involve the cardiovascular and central nervous systems (**Table 12**).

Should a toxic reaction or overdose from LA occur, several treatment options exist for the practitioner. One option for treating minimal to moderate LA overdose is to give a reversal agent. OraVerse (phentolamine) is a short-acting alpha blocker. It reverses the vasoconstrictor effect and shortens the LA duration. It is only for use with vasoconstrictor-containing LAs. It is packaged as 1.7 mg in a 1.8 mL cartridge, and the maximum dose is two cartridges. For moderate or high overdose as the symptoms worsen, Intralipid™ 20% IV emulsion can be administered. This drug increases the concentration of serum proteins available for binding the LA. Usual dosing is to administer 1 mL/kg over 1 min and to repeat twice more at 3- to 5-min intervals. Then (or sooner if stability is restored), the practitioner can convert to an infusion at a rate of 0.25 mL/kg/min, continuing until hemodynamic stability is restored. As a last resort, emergency dialysis can be considered.

4.18. Epinephrine

Lidocaine remains the most common local anesthetic medication administered in OMFS and dental offices; therefore, a deeper review of this medication, its properties, and its toxicity is warranted. **Table 13** lists adult dosages for the most common preparations of lidocaine in dental carpules (2% solutions, 1.7 mL total volume/carpule). Most OMSs prefer to use the lidocaine preparation with epinephrine due to its favorable vasoconstrictive properties. A 1:100,000 concentration of epinephrine translates to 0.01 mg/mL or 0.017 mg/carpule. The American Heart Association regards no more than 0.04 mg epinephrine generally as safe for patients with uncontrolled/poorly controlled hypertension or a significant cardiac history. This, however, is based more on anecdotal rather than empiric evidence as injection variables such as the time frame over which the medication is administered or whether the injection was given intravascular become important factors.

Agent	Cartridge size (mg)	Max dose (mg/kg)	Max dose (mg/lb)	Max dose (mg)
2% lidocaine	34	4.5	2	300
2% lidocaine w/1:100k epi	34	7	3.3	500

Maximum dosages are based on an adult weight of 150 lb or 70 kg and taken from the manufacturer (Astra).

Table 13. Adult dosages for lidocaine as commonly used in OMFS practice

Contrary to popular belief, epinephrine will not alter mean arterial pressure as α vasoconstriction is balanced by β dilation. Epinephrine will, however, accelerate heart rate, which will *increase* myocardial oxygen demand secondary to the tachycardia and *decrease* oxygen supply secondary to decreased diastolic fill time and decreased diastolic coronary perfusion time. Since most patients with known coronary artery diseases are stented, the epinephrine-induced tachycardia is only an issue with heart failure and other structural heart diseases. Epinephrine is direct acting and therefore has no interaction with monoamine oxidase inhibitors. It may increase blood pressure when given to patients taking tricyclic antidepressants, and will increase blood pressure and decrease heart rate when used in patients taking non-selective β blockers.

4.19. Causes and clinical manifestations of local anesthetic (LA) toxicity

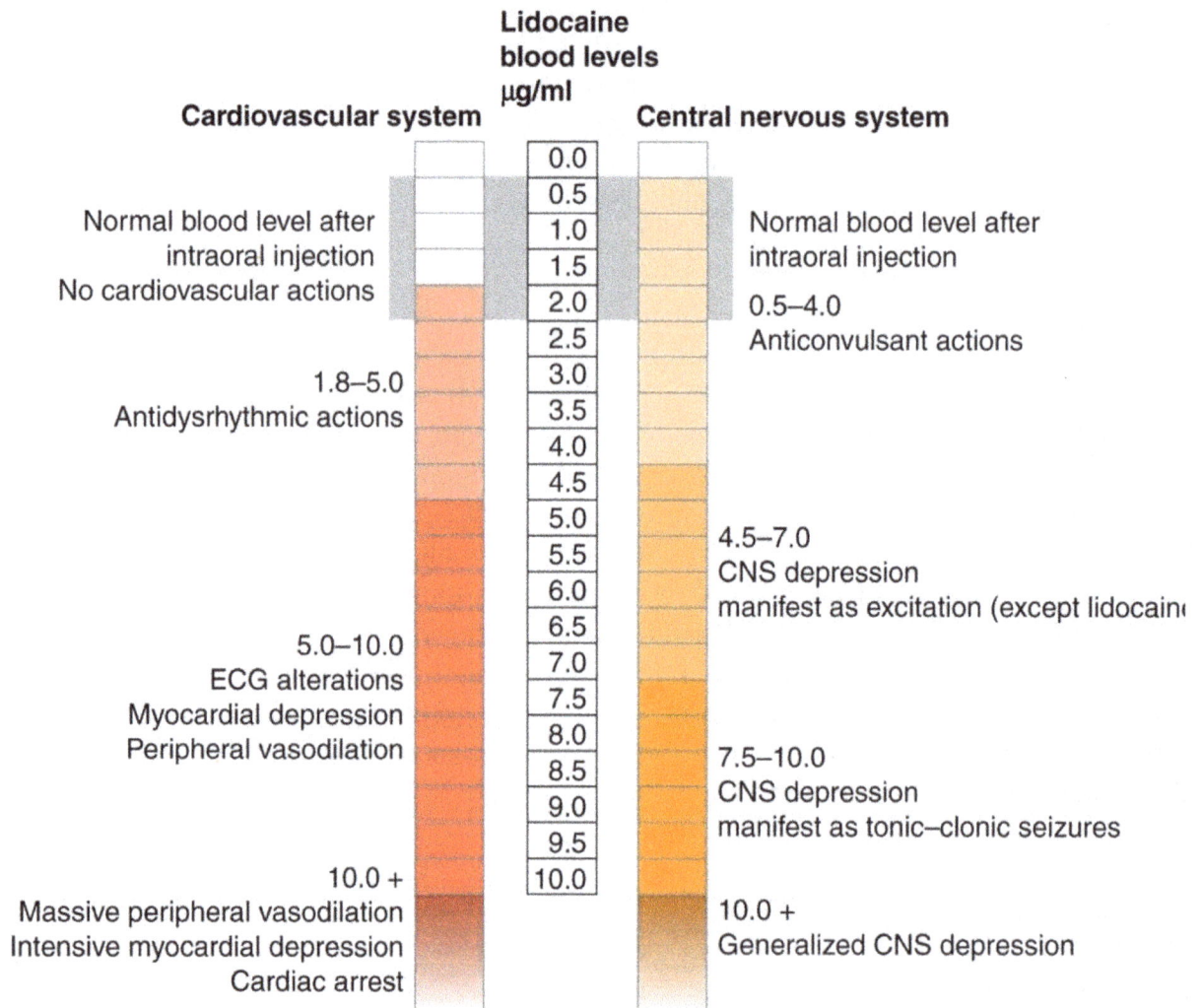

Cardiovascular system	Lidocaine blood levels μg/ml	Central nervous system
	0.0	
	0.5	
Normal blood level after	1.0	Normal blood level after
intraoral injection	1.5	intraoral injection
No cardiovascular actions	2.0	0.5–4.0
	2.5	Anticonvulsant actions
	3.0	
1.8–5.0	3.5	
Antidysrhythmic actions	4.0	
	4.5	
	5.0	
	5.5	4.5–7.0
	6.0	CNS depression
	6.5	manifest as excitation (except lidocaine
5.0–10.0	7.0	
ECG alterations	7.5	
Myocardial depression	8.0	
Peripheral vasodilation	8.5	7.5–10.0
	9.0	CNS depression
	9.5	manifest as tonic–clonic seizures
10.0 +	10.0	
Massive peripheral vasodilation		10.0 +
Intensive myocardial depression		Generalized CNS depression
Cardiac arrest		

Table 14. Local anesthetic (Lidocaine) blood levels and their actions on cardiovascular and central nervous systems [31].

Elevated plasma levels of the anesthetic could lead to local anesthetic toxicity. This may be caused by an inadvertent intravascular injection or by iatrogenically violating the maximum (mg/kg) dose. Geriatric and pediatric patients are at greatest risks for LA toxicity. Older patients generally metabolize drugs at a slower rate. A geriatric patient who takes multiple medications may experience adverse drug reactions when lidocaine is administered. Cimetidine, a histamine H_2-receptor antagonist, inhibits the hepatic oxidative enzymes (P-450) needed for metabolism, thereby allowing lidocaine to accumulate in the circulating blood. This adverse reaction is seen only with cimetidine and not with other H_2-receptor antagonists. Propranolol, a beta-adrenergic blocker, can reduce both hepatic blood flow and lidocaine clearance. Toxic reaction could result if high doses of lidocaine are given to patients taking either or both of these medications. A possible additive adverse drug reaction exists with the administration of LAs and opioids in the geriatric and pediatric populations as well. Opioids (fentanyl, meperidine, and morphine) may cause an amide LA additive effect because of their similar chemical structures (both are basic lipophilic amines) and a first-pass pulmonary effect. The lungs may serve as a reservoir for these drugs with a subsequent release back into the system.

4.20. Lidocaine toxicity and cardiovascular effects

Lidocaine has a depressive effect on the myocardium (**Table 14**). Toxic doses of lidocaine cause sinus bradycardia because lidocaine increases the effective refractory period relative to the action potential duration and decreases cardiac automaticity. If a very high dose has been administered, impaired cardiac contractibility, arteriolar dilation, profound hypotension, and circulatory collapse can result [32].

4.21. Lidocaine toxicity and central nervous system (CNS) effects

Lidocaine usually has a sedative effect on the brain (**Table 14**). Initially, lidocaine toxicity depresses brain function in the form of drowsiness and slurred speech. Its effects may progress to unconsciousness and even coma [33].

4.22. Cardiovascular *actions* of lidocaine

Lidocaine is frequently used in the management of various ventricular dysrhythmias, especially ventricular extrasystole (premature ventricular contractions) and ventricular tachycardia. Alterations occur in the myocardium as blood levels of lidocaine increase. In general, the minimal effective blood level of lidocaine for antidysrhythmic activity is 1.8 (μg/mL). In the range from approximately 2–5 (μg/mL), the actions of lidocaine on the myocardium consist only of electrophysiological changes. These include a prolongation or abolition of the slow phase of depolarization during diastole in Purkinje fibers and a shortening of the action potential duration of the effective refractory period. At this therapeutic level, no alterations in myocardial contractility, diastolic volume, intraventricular pressure, or cardiac output are evident. Both the healthy and diseased myocardia tolerate mildly elevated blood levels of lidocaine without deleterious effects. When used to treat dysrhythmias, lidocaine is administered intravenously in a 50–100-mg bolus (1.0–1.5 mg/kg). Overdose is a potential concern, but the generous benefit-to-risk ratio allows for the judicious use of IV lidocaine. Further elevation of the lidocaine blood level (5–10 μg/mL) produces a prolongation of conduction time through various portions of the heart and an increase in the diastolic threshold. This may be noted on the ECG as an increased P-R interval and QRS duration as well as sinus bradycardia. In addition, decreased myocardial contractility, increased diastolic volume, decreased intraventricular pressure, and decreased cardiac output become evident. Peripheral vascular effects observed at this level include vasodilation, which produces a decrease in blood pressure and occurs as a result of the direct relaxant effect of lidocaine on peripheral vascular smooth muscle. Further increases in blood levels of lidocaine (>10 µg/mL) lead to an accentuation of the electrophysiological and hemodynamic effects such as massive peripheral vasodilation, marked decrease in myocardial contractility, and slowed heart rate, which may ultimately result in cardiac arrest.

4.23. Risk factors for lidocaine toxicity

Older age (>60) and pediatric patients are susceptible to lidocaine overdose and toxicity reactions. Those with decreased body weight, along with patients with medical comorbidities such as congestive heart failure, acute MI, and decreased hepatic function are also at risk. Continued risk includes patients with concomitant use of drugs decreasing P-450 activity (such as cimetidine) that triggers lidocaine accumulation in the blood. Like with other LAs, a possible additive adverse drug reaction exists with administration of lidocaine and opioids in the geriatric and pediatric populations [33].

4.24. Management of mild lidocaine overdose with rapid onset

An overdose in which signs and symptoms develop within 5–10 min following drug administration is considered rapid in onset (**Table 15**). Possible causes include intravascular injection, unusually rapid absorption, or administration of a large total dose. If clinical manifestations do not progress beyond mild central nervous system excitation and consciousness is retained, significant and definitive care is not necessary. The local anesthetic undergoes redistribution and biotransformation, with the blood level falling below the overdose level in a relatively short time.

Method of overdose	Likelihood of occurrence	Onset of signs and symptoms	Intensity of signs and symptoms	Duration	Primary prevention	Drug
Too large of a dose given	Most common	5–30 min	Gradual onset w/ increased intensity; may prove severe	5–30 min	Administer minimal doses	Amides; esters rarely

Table 15. Most common form of local anesthetic overdose

4.25. Toxicity reversal

Increasing evidence suggests that the intravenous (IV) infusion of lipid emulsions can reverse the cardiac and neurologic effects of local-anesthetic toxicity [32]. Although no blinded studies have so far been conducted in humans, studies in animal models and multiple case reports in human patients have shown favorable results. Indeed, case reports support the early use of lipid emulsion at the first sign of arrhythmia, prolonged seizure activity, or rapid progression of toxic manifestations in patients with suspected local anesthetic toxicity. Intralipid™ 20% emulsion IV may be administered at 1 mL/kg over 1 min. This is to be repeated twice more at

3- to 5-min intervals. Then (or sooner if stability is restored), convert to an infusion at a rate of 0.25 mL/kg/min, continuing until hemodynamic stability is restored. This increases the concentration of serum protein available for binding to lidocaine. As a last resort, the practitioner can consider emergency hemodialysis.

4.26. Stable versus unstable/symptomatic bradycardia

Bradycardia is defined as any rhythm disorder with a HR < 60 beats per minute (bpm). Stable bradycardia can be a normal non-emergent rhythm. For instance, well-trained athletes may have a normal HR < 60 bpm. Symptomatic bradycardia is defined as a rate that is <60 bpm that elicits signs (hypotension, congestive heart failure, myocardial infarction, and hypoxia) and symptoms (chest pain, shortness of breath, decreased level of consciousness). Symptomatic bradycardia will usually manifest with HR < 50 bpm.

4.27. Management of unstable/symptomatic bradycardia with pulse (HR < 50 and inadequate for clinical condition) [34]:

Includes following a treatment protocol resembling this algorithm:

- Establish a secure airway

- Obtain intravenous (IV) access

- Administer oxygen

- Monitor blood pressure and rhythm

- Administer atropine 0.5 mg via IV q3–5 min, maximum 3 mg

- Consider transcutaneous pacing, or

- Consider dopamine 2–10 μg/kg/min, or

- Consider epinephrine 2–10 μg/min, or

- Consider isoproterenol 2–10 μg/min

4.28. Anesthetic preparation

Though significant anesthetic complications in the OMFS office are rare, an American Society of Anesthesiology closed claims analysis reported that up to 80% of anesthetic mishaps were attributable to human error [35] Practitioners and their staff may not be fluent in management of these situations unless they routinely practice emergency scenarios and have made regular preparations for such events. Emergency management preparation must consist of the following components: thinking about the emergency (pathophysiology of the event and decision making), doing (taking responsibility), and interacting (communicating to staff and auxiliary personnel and maintaining leadership). This preparation can be enhanced by staging repeated and simulated rehearsals within the OMFS office.

For most OMSs, anesthetic management is routine, but uncertainties and emergencies are bound to arise. The OMFS office must develop, implement, and practice protocols to optimize patient care and emergency management that balances practicality with the premises of "do no harm" and "always be prepared."

5. Conclusion

Deep sedation and general anesthesia can be safely administered in the OMFS office. Optimization of patient care requires appropriate patient selection, thorough understanding of medical comorbidities and body systems, selection of appropriate anesthetic agents for the individual being treated, utilization of appropriate anesthetic monitoring, and a well-trained office anesthesia team. Achieving a highly trained team requires emergency management preparation that helps foster decision making in intense circumstances, develops leadership, formulates communication strategies, and perfects task management. Furthermore, the privilege and ability to provide patient care under anesthesia is a continuum that extends beyond this initial training. Safe anesthetic care can be provided, but doing so requires effort that entails constant maintenance of current knowledge, preparation, and teamwork.

Author details

Jeffrey A. Elo[1,2*] and Ho-Hyun Sun[3]

*Address all correspondence to: jelo@westernu.edu

1 Division of Oral and Maxillofacial Surgery, Western University of Health Sciences College of Dental Medicine, Pomona, California, USA

2 Department of Oral and Maxillofacial Surgery, Loma Linda University Medical Center, Loma Linda, California, USA

3 Western University of Health Sciences College of Dental Medicine, Pomona, California, USA

References

[1] D'Eramo EM, Bontempi WJ, Howard JB. Anesthesia morbidity and mortality experience among Massachusetts oral and maxillofacial surgeons. J Oral Maxillofac Surg. 2008;66(12):2421–2433.

[2] D'Eramo EM, Bookless SJ, Howard JB. Adverse events with outpatient anesthesia in Massachusetts. J Oral Maxillofac Surg. 2003;61(7):793–800.

[3] Metzner J, Posner KL, Domino KB. The risk and safety of anesthesia at remote locations: the US closed claims analysis. Cur Opin Anaesthesiol. 2009;22:502–508.

[4] Rodgers SF, Rodgers MS. Safety of intravenous sedation administered by the operating oral surgeon: the second 7 years of office practice. J Oral Maxillofac Surg. 2011;69(10): 2525–2529.

[5] Weaver JM. Comparison of morbidity of outpatient general anesthesia administered by the intravenous or inhalation route. J Oral Maxillofac Surg. 1998;56(9):1038–1039.

[6] Braidy HF, Singh P, Ziccardi VB. Safety of deep sedation in an urban oral and maxillofacial surgery training program. J Oral Maxillofac Surg. 2011;69(8):2112–2119.

[7] Hunter MJ, Molinaro AM. Morbidity and mortality with outpatient anesthesia: the experience of a residency training program. J Oral Maxillofac Surg. 1997;55(7):684–687.

[8] Lytle JJ. Morbidity and mortality with outpatient anesthesia: the experience of a residency training program. J Oral Maxillofac Surg. 1997;55(7):687–688.

[9] http://www.aaoms.org/images/uploads/pdfs/parcare_assessment.pdf.

[10] American Society of Anesthesiologists. Practice guidelines for preoperative fasting and the use of pharmacologic agents to reduce the risk of pulmonary aspiration: application to healthy patients undergoing elective procedures. Anesthesiology. 2011;114:495.

[11] Fleisher LE, Beckman JA, Brown KA, et al. ACC/AHA 2007 Guidelines on perioperative cardiovascular evaluation and care for noncardiac surgery: executive summary: a report of the American College of Cardiology/American Heart Association Task Force on Practice Guidelines (Writing committee to revise the 2002 guidelines on perioperative cardiovascular evaluation for noncardiac surgery). Circulation. 2007;116:1971–1996.

[12] Jetté M, Sidney K, Blümchen G. Metabolic equivalents (METS) in exercise testing, exercise prescription, and evaluation of functional capacity. Clin Cardiol. 1990;13(8): 555–565.

[13] Lee TH, Marcantonio ER, Mangione CM, et al. Derivation and prospective validation of a simple index for prediction of cardiac risk of major noncardiac surgery. Circulation. 1999;100:1043–1049.

[14] Arozullah AM, Conde MV, Lawrence VA. Preoperative evaluation for postoperative pulmonary complications. Med Clin North Am. 2003;87(1):153–173.

[15] Caplan RA, Posner KL, Ward RJ, Cheney FW. Adverse respiratory events in anesthesia: a closed claims analysis. Anesthesiology. 1990;72:828–833.

[16] Lan CK, Rose MW. Perioperative management of obstructive sleep apnea. Sleep Med Clin. 2006;1(4):541–548.

[17] Pawlik MT, Hansen E, Waldhauser D, et al. Clonidine premedication in patients with sleep apnea syndrome: a randomized, double-blind, placebo-controlled study. Anesth Analg. 2005;101(5):1374–1380.

[18] Cheung AH, Wong LM. Surgical infections in patients with chronic renal failure. Infect Dis Clin North Am. 2001;15(3):775–796.

[19] Hoste EA, De Waele JJ. Physiologic consequences of acute renal failure on the critically ill. Crit Care Clin. 2005;21(2):251–260.

[20] Clement S, Braithwaite SS, Magee MF, et al. Management of diabetes and hyperglycemia in hospitals. Diabetes Care. 2004;27:553–591.

[21] Furnary AP, Zerr KJ, Grunkemeier GL, Starr A. Continuous intravenous insulin infusion reduces the incidence of deep sternal wound infection in diabetic patients after cardiac surgical procedures. Ann Thorac Surg. 1999;67(2):352–360.

[22] Furnary AP, Gao G, Grunkemeier GL, et al. Continuous insulin infusion reduces mortality in patients with diabetes undergoing coronary artery bypass grafting. J Thorac Cardiovasc Surg. 2003;125:1007–1021.

[23] Pomposelli JJ, Baxter JK III, Babineau TJ, et al. Early postoperative glucose control predicts nosocomial infection rates in diabetic patients. J Parenter Enteral Nutr. 1998;22:77–81.

[24] Van den Berghe G, Wouters P, Weekers F, et al. Intensive insulin therapy in critically ill patients. N Engl J Med. 2001;345:1359–1367.

[25] Adams VHA. The mechanisms of action of ketamine. Anaesthes Reanim. 1998;23(3):60–63.

[26] Bowdle TA, Radan AD, Cowley DS, Kharasch ED, Strassman RJ, Roy-Byrne PP. Psychedelic effects of ketamine in healthy volunteers: relationship to steady-state plasma concentrations. Anesthesiology. 1998;88(1):82–88.

[27] Clements JA, Nimo WS, Grant IS. Bioavailability, pharmacokinetics and analgesic activity of ketamine in humans. J Pharm Sci. 1982;71(5):539–542.

[28] Adler CM, Goldberg TE, Malhotra AK, Pickar D, Breier A. Effects of ketamine on thought disorder, working memory, and semantic memory in healthy volunteers. Biol Psychiat. 1998;43(11):811–816.

[29] Gengo F, Gabos C, Miller JK. The pharmacodynamics of diphenhydramine-induced drowsiness and changes in mental performances. Clin Pharmacol Ther. 1989;45:15–21.

[30] Gengo FM, Manning C. A review of the effects of antihistamines on mental processes related to automobile driving. J Allergy Clin Immunol. 1990;86:1034–1039.

[31] Malamed SF. Handbook of local anesthesia, 5 ed., St. Louis, Mosby, 2004.

[32] Neal JM, Mulroy MF, Weinberg GL. American Society of Regional Anesthesia and Pain Medicine checklist for managing local anesthetic systemic toxicity: 2012 version. Reg Anesth Pain Med. 2012;37:16–18.

[33] Bursell B, Ratzan RM, Smally AJ. Lidocaine toxicity misinterpreted as a stroke. West J Emerg Med. 2009;10:292–294.

[34] ACLS 2010 Guidelines, Circ. 2010;122(Suppl 3):S729.

[35] Cooper J, Newbower R, Long C, McPeek B. Preventable anesthesia mishaps: a study of human factors. Qual Saf Health Care. 2002;11(3):277–282.

7

Cranial Nerves and Nerve Surgery in the Oral and Maxillofacial Region

Shahram Nazerani and Tina Nazerani

Abstract

The head and neck surgeon is confronted with cranial nerves in the course of operations and he or she must know the anatomy and the ways to treat complications should they happen. In this chapter we focus on the subject of cranial nerves and begin with the history and anatomy and then to individual nerves and maladies of these nerves and complications of surgical procedures involving these nerves.

Keywords: cranial nerves, cranial nerve disorders, cranial nerve surgery, nerve repair, nerve transfer

1. Introduction

Ancient Egyptian mummification artisans had no consideration for the brain; the internal organs such as the liver, intestines, lung, and heart were preserved in separate jars; they broke the skull bone through the nose with a tool like a hook and a tool to blend lift the brain and then allowed it to drain out the nose or flushed it out with water. The Egyptians thought the heart was the site of bravery and gave no importance to the brain for afterlife preservation (**Figure 1**).

The history regarding exploration of the cranial nerves and their anatomy is ancient. Galen's classification of the cranial nerves, excluding the olfactory nerve, was composed of seven pairs; the sixth pair included the glossopharyngeal, vagus, and accessory nerves all traveling through the jugular foramen [1].

The cranial nerves were essentially identified and numbered based on the opening through which they exited the skull base. Our knowledge of the cranial nerves grew more clearly by medieval Middle Eastern and European scholars such as Rhazes, Avicenna, Jorjani, Mundinus, Benedetti, Achillini, Massa, and Berengario deCarpi [2].

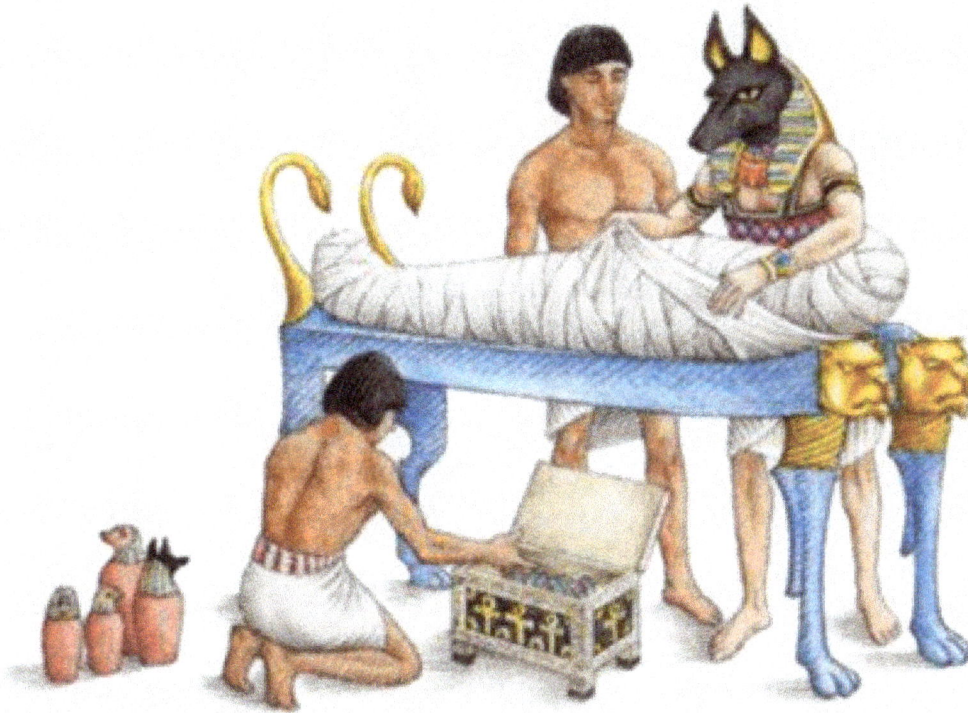

Figure 1. Mummification process with internal organs set aside in jars.

Italian anatomists in the fourteenth and fifteenth centuries identified the olfactory nerve as a cranial nerve. The work of these anatomists laid the foundation for the doctoral thesis of the German anatomist Samuel Sömmerring (1755–1830 AD), who in 1778 classified the 12 cranial nerves as we recognize them today [3, 4]. In his thesis, Sömmerring made no meaningful anatomical discoveries, and his classification is essentially no less different from previous anatomists. Nonetheless, the Sömmerring system was rapidly adopted across continental Europe, although it was only slowly accepted in England [5].

2. Anatomy and naming of the cranial nerves

The cranial nerve nomenclature is an ordinal system introduced presumably by Galen, by which the nerves are named by their location on the undersurface of the brain, this system has stood the test of time and has not been changed during the ages, although the olfactory nerve has been mentioned even before Galen's ordinal classification. Modern anatomists argue that the olfactory and optic nerves are tracts and not true cranial nerves and should be removed from the "twelve-nerve" classification system [5]. To memorize these nerves, several mnemonics have been devised (**Figure 2**).

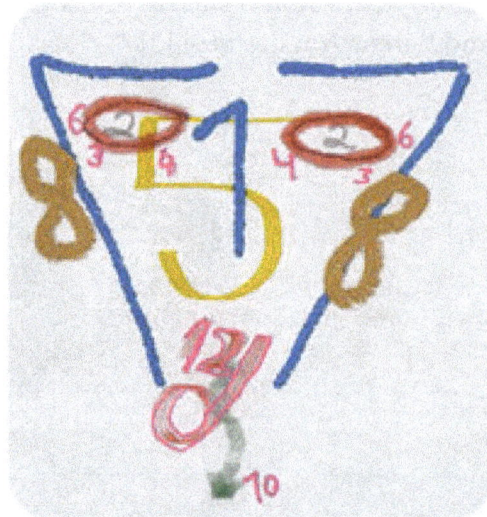

Figure 2. A mnemonic of the cranial nerves.

Galen's classification of cranial nerves is depicted below; he identified seven pairs but he assigned no names to them. The modern classification is shown below, Galen identified seven pairs of nerves, and the interesting point is that the old scholars saw the brain as a whole and not two hemispheres of an organ.

Modern classification:

I. Olfactory nerve

II. Optic nerve

III. Oculomotor nerve

IV. Trochlear nerve

V. Trigeminal nerve

VI. Abducens nerve

VII. Facial nerve

VIII. Vestibulocochlear nerve

IX. Glossopharyngeal nerve

X. Vagus nerve

XI. Accessory nerve

XII. Hypoglossal nerve

3. Surgical importance of cranial nerves

There are 12 cranial nerves, but only some of the nerve problems were identified and reported in the early ages. Of the 12 cranial nerves, the trigeminal and facial nerves have been under more scrutiny: the trigeminal due to its excruciating pain and the facial nerve due to its characteristic facial disfigurement in nerve palsy (**Figure 3**).

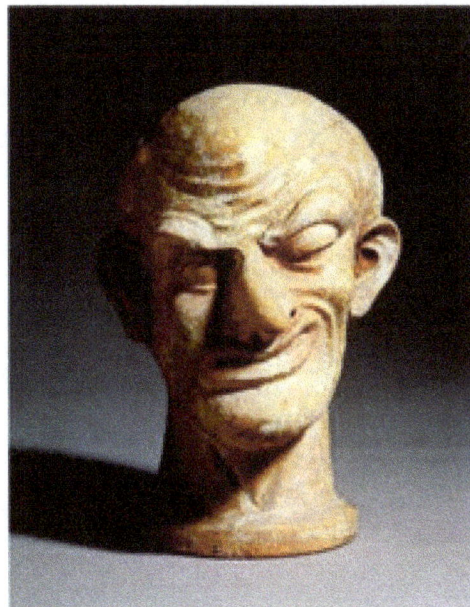

Figure 3. A sculpture of facial palsy.

Other cranial nerves are usually noticed when traumatized, involved in tumoral conditions or injured during an operation.

Multiple cranial nerves are usually involved in procedures such as carotid endarterectomy, anesthesia, and cancer surgery. In a review article, Thiruvenkatarajan et al. investigated cranial nerve injury (CNI) during anesthesia and they found that cranial nerve injuries are unusual complications of supraglottic airway use. Branches of the trigeminal (V), glossopharyngeal (IX), vagus (X), and hypoglossal (XII) nerves may be injured. Lingual nerve (LN) injury was the most commonly reported, followed by recurrent laryngeal, hypoglossal, glossopharyngeal, inferior alveolar, and infraorbital. The culprit is usually poor technique and inappropriate pressure on the nerves due to wrong size or misplacement or overinflation of the cuff. Injury to the recurrent laryngeal nerve (RLN) is usually more long lasting than other nerves involved [6]. In a multicenter prospective study, Fokkema et al. investigated the prevalence of CNI in carotid endarterectomy; 6878 patients were included for analyses. CNI rate at discharge was 5.6%. Sixty patients (0.7%) had more than one nerve affected. The hypoglossal nerve was most frequently involved (2.7%), followed by the facial (1.9%), the vagus (0.7%), and the glosso-pharyngeal (0.5%) nerve. The vast majority of these CNIs were transient; only 47 patients (0.7%) had a persistent CNI at their follow-up visit [7]. Isolated cranial nerve injuries are herein with special attention to the nerves more prone to injury during maxillofacial surgery.

3.1. The olfactory nerve

The first cranial nerve is composed of receptor neurons which connect the nasal cavity to the brain (**Figure 4**). The nerve dendrites reside in the nasal cavity on the apical side and the axons pass through the cribriform plate of the skull into the olfactory area of the brain [8].

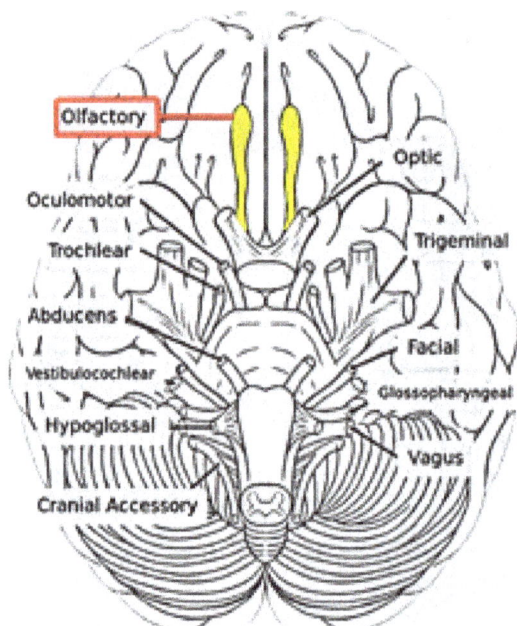

Figure 4. Skull base schematic diagram and the olfactory nerve marked in yellow.

Esthesioneuroblastoma (ENB) is a rare malignant neoplasm arising from the olfactory neuroepithelium. ENB constitutes only 3% of all malignant intranasal neoplasms. Because of the rarity, the number of patients of ENB treated in individual departments is small. Most of these patients present in locally advanced stages and require multimodality surgery, chemotherapy, and radiotherapy [9]. Impairment of smell may occur following injury to any portion of the olfactory tract, from the nasal cavity to brain. A thorough understanding of the anatomy and pathophysiology combined with comprehensively obtained history, physical exam, olfactory testing, and neuroimaging may help to identify the mechanism of dysfunction and suggest possible treatments. Although most olfactory deficits are neuronal mediated and therefore currently unable to be corrected, promising technology may provide novel treatment options for those most affected. Until that day, patient counseling with compensatory strategies and reassurance is essential in this unique and challenging patient population [10].

3.2. Optic nerve

Optic nerve injury may have several etiologies such as tumor, trauma, and inflammation, but in the context of maxillofacial surgery, trauma to the optic nerve is the most important (**Figure 5**); two types of trauma to the optic nerve are seen, primary and secondary; injury to the nerve fibers and/or vascular supply can be due to direct injury at the time of trauma or secondary as the result of compromised blood supply to the nerve.

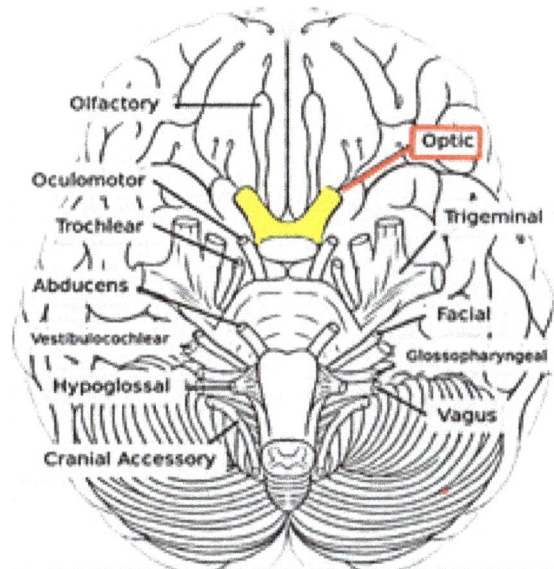

Figure 5. Optic nerve marked in yellow.

3.3. Oculomotor nerve

Injuries to the oculomotor nerve present with nerve palsy manifestations (**Figure 6**); the etiologies can be sellar chordoma, odontogenic abscess, non-aneurysmal subarachnoid hemorrhage, polycythemia, sphenoiditis, brucellosis, interpeduncular fossa lipoma, metastatic cancer, and blood and lymph cancers. Surgical options are correction of nerve palsy, i.e., strabismus surgery. New globe fixation procedures may include fixation to the medial orbital wall, apically based orbital bone periosteal flap fixation, and the suture/T-plate anchoring platform technique [11].

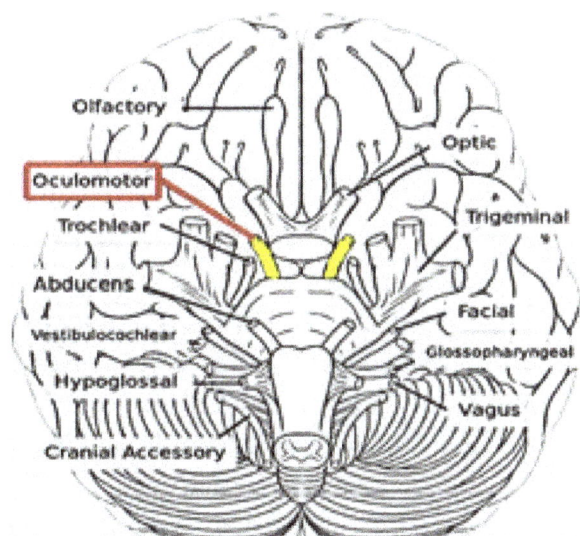

Figure 6. The third cranial nerve marked in yellow.

3.4. Trochlear nerve

The trochlear nerve originates from the trochlear nuclei in the caudal midbrain (**Figure 7**) and carries primarily motor fibers destined for the superior oblique muscle; the nerve may be encountered in many areas such as the supracerebellar, middle cranial fossa, parasellar, and orbital regions. This nerve was the last cranial nerve found, due its small size and lack of fixation techniques in the earlier periods of anatomical studies. Trauma, tumors, viral infection, and surgery can all injure this nerve with impaired eyeball movement.

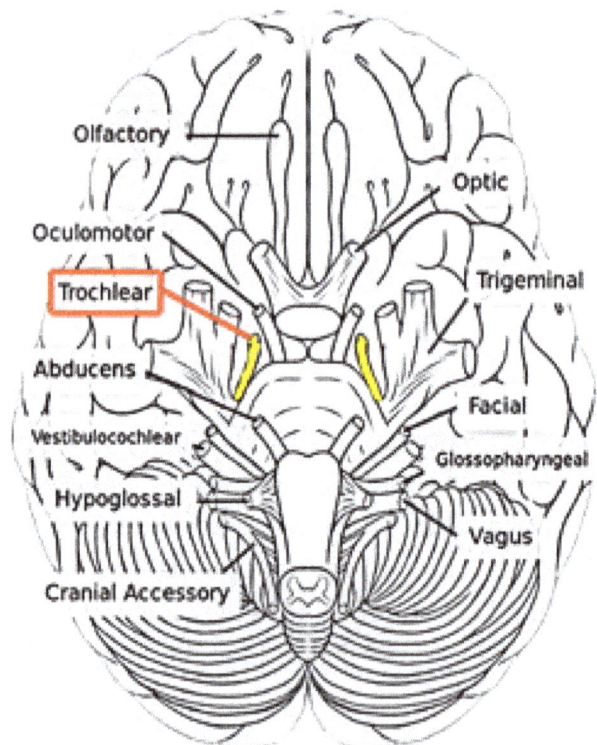

Figure 7. The fourth cranial nerve seen from undersurface of the brain.

3.5. Trigeminal nerve

The trigeminal nerve is the largest and most complex of the 12 cranial nerves (**Figure 8**). The three branches of the trigeminal nerve (the ophthalmic, maxillary, and mandibular branches exit the skull through three separate foramina, namely, the superior orbital fissure, the foramen rotundum, and the foramen ovale, respectively). The mandibular branch had mixed sensory and motor neurons and of all the branches lingual and inferior alveolar are more prone to injury during maxillofacial operations. Injury to the LN and/or inferior alveolar nerve (IAN) is a known complication associated with several oral and maxillofacial surgical procedures. Bagheri et al. in a retrospective study have shown that microsurgical repair of LN and IAN injury has the best chance of successful restoration of acceptable neurosensory function if done within 9 months of the injury. As in all other nerves, the likelihood of recovery decreases progressively when the repair is done more than 9 months after injury [12].

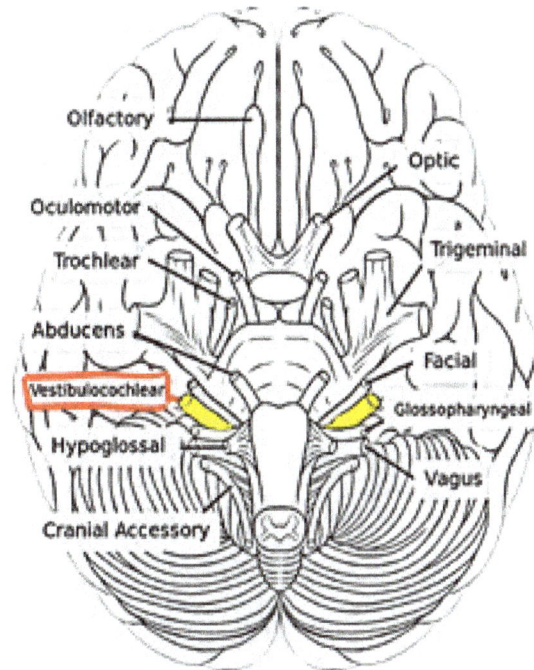

Figure 8. The fifth cranial nerve, the largest cranial nerve.

3.6. Abducens nerve

The sixth cranial nerve is a motor nerve with diplopia as its presenting symptom when injured (**Figure 9**). Binocular diplopia occurs from misalignment of the eyes. The fixation object is imaged onto the fovea of one eye and a non-foveal region of the misaligned eye, creating diplopia. The nerve can be injured in head trauma, autoimmune diseases, and several other conditions. Treatment options include ocular occlusion, mono-vision optical correction, prism glasses, strabismus surgery, and chemo-denervation.

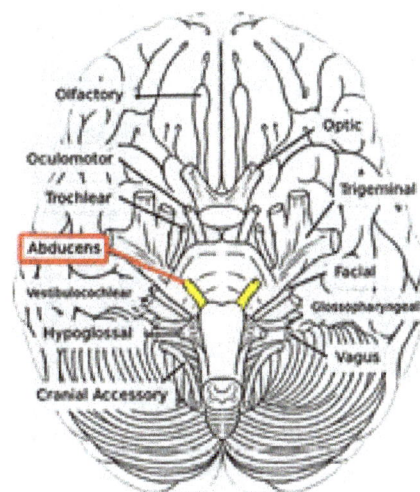

Figure 9. The sixth cranial nerve.

3.7. Facial nerve

Facial nerve paralysis involves orifice control for the eye, nose, and mouth, as well as facial expression (**Figure 10**). The lack of orifice control for the eye can lead to corneal exposure, keratopathy, and potential visual loss. The orifice control relating to the nose can cause difficulties in breathing with lack of normal opening of the involved nostril.

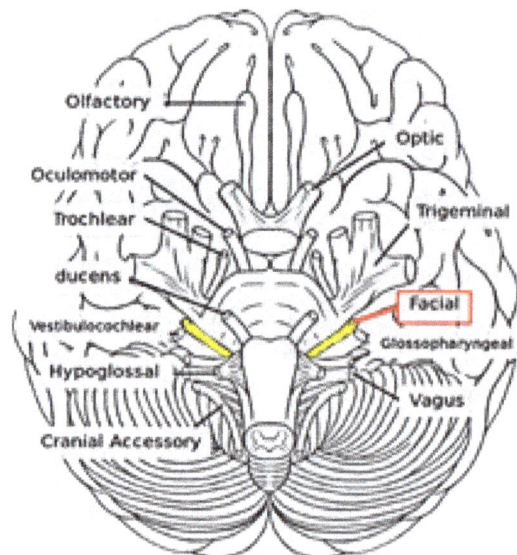

Figure 10. The seventh cranial nerve.

The lack of orifice control for the mouth can affect the symmetry of the face with drooping of the involved side, as well as problems related to speech, chewing, and oral competence leading to drooling. In some cases, the lack of dental protection can lead to dental decay. Some partial facial palsies are seen as attractive (**Figure 11**).

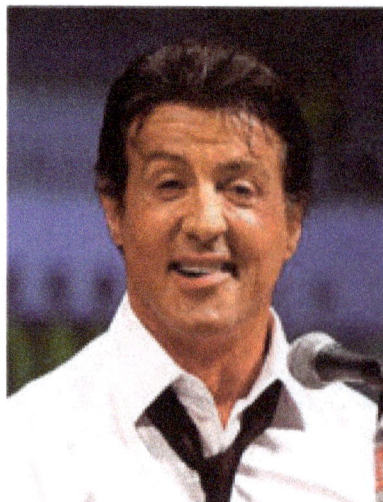

Figure 11. Sylvester Stallone with his "trademark smile."

The mimetic function, however, of the facial nerve is critical for social interactions. Nonverbal communication is conveyed by facial expression and is essential for normal interpersonal interactions. A smile invokes a smile in others and conveys feelings that cannot be transmitted in any other way. Consequently, a spontaneous dynamic smile is critical for personal interactions. Treatment modalities in facial paralysis and associated movement disorders are numerous and vary based on individual needs and preferences.

3.7.1. Congenital facial paralysis

The anatomical presentation of developmental facial paralysis can be summarized into four categories:

1. Aplasia or hypoplasia of cranial nerve nuclei

2. Nuclear agenesis

3. Peripheral nerve abnormalities

4. Primary myopathy [13]

3.7.2. Acquired facial paralysis

Three stages of facial nerve paralysis are acute, intermediate, and chronic; the treatment modalities are discussed below.

3.7.3. Acute facial paralysis

Identifiable causes of acute paralysis are treated with appropriate medical therapy, following proper identification of the cause. In rare instances, surgical intervention may be necessary to control infection and/or swelling around the facial nerve. In trauma or resection of cancer invading the facial nerve, several reconstructive options are available. These minimize the sequelae of paralysis, optimize immediate patient recovery, and promote the return of facial nerve function.

3.7.4. Intermediate facial paralysis

During this stage (3 weeks to 2 years), facial nerve recovery is monitored with serial electrophysiological studies, which provide useful prognostic data. In a setting of poorly recovering facial nerve, several procedures can be considered to restore facial appearance and rehabilitate function around the eye and mouth. In the early stages gold weight placement to aid upper eyelid closure (lagophthalmos) and static sling suspension of the midface and lip can be performed with minimal associated downtime. Lagophthalmus (**Figures 12** and **13**) can be treated by a range of techniques, including tarsorrhaphy, facial slings, and canthopexies. Gold plates provide a solution for temporary or permanent lagophthalmos resulting from facial paralysis. Amer et al. studied the use of gold plates in two different positions in the upper lids.

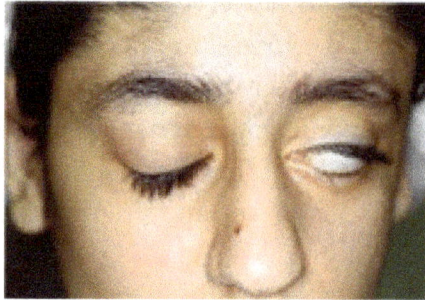

Figure 12. Bell's palsy and lagophthalmos.

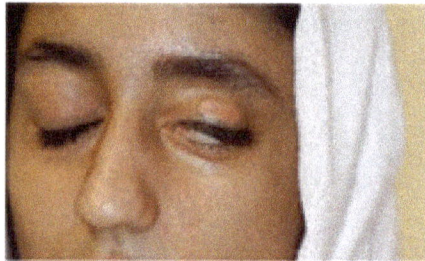

Figure 13. Gold plate inserted, but is not esthetically appealing.

They concluded that gold plate insertion at a higher than usual place of insertion can reduce the drawbacks of lower placement such as "plate show," thinning of the skin over the plate [14].

These procedures do not interfere with the recovering facial nerve. In the later stages, if the facial nerve continues to display poor recovery on EMG, consideration is given to nerve transfer procedures designed to maintain neurological input of facial muscles. A graft from a nearby nerve, most commonly the hypoglossal, can provide such input. Terzis and Karypidis show that cross-facial nerve grafting and concomitant mini-hypoglossal transfer are the procedures that yield higher improvement in blink scores and ratios compared with the rest of the dynamic procedures. Direct orbicularis oculi muscle neurotization achieves a fair blink improvement [15].

3.7.5. Chronic facial paralysis

3.7.5.1. Paralysis

Management of chronic facial paralysis, more than two years, depends on numerous factors, including patient preferences, age, and desires. Medical considerations may also limit the available procedures. Reconstructive options range from static suspensions to reanimate via muscle transfer to the paralyzed side.

Static slings such as native fascia (5) or permanent sutures (6) are the easiest methods in facial reanimation. These slings hold the paralyzed side in midline and help hold the lips and prevent drooling to a degree. Static slings relax and descend over time, thus potentially requiring additional tightening [16, 17] (**Figures 14–18**).

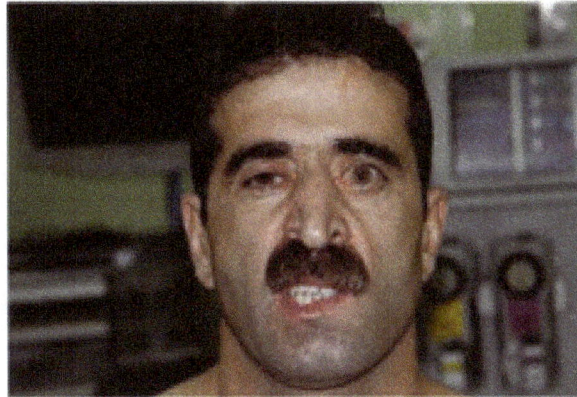

Figure 14. Chronic Bell's palsy, first-stage sural nerve transfer already done.

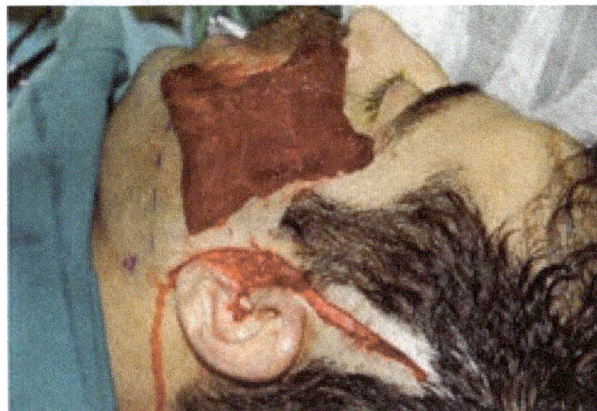

Figure 15. Gracilis muscle bisected and ready for insertion.

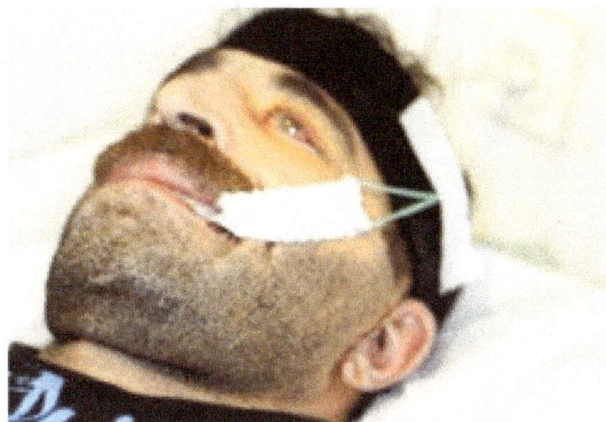

Figure 16. Two months after the operation and the static splint for maintaining the muscle suture.

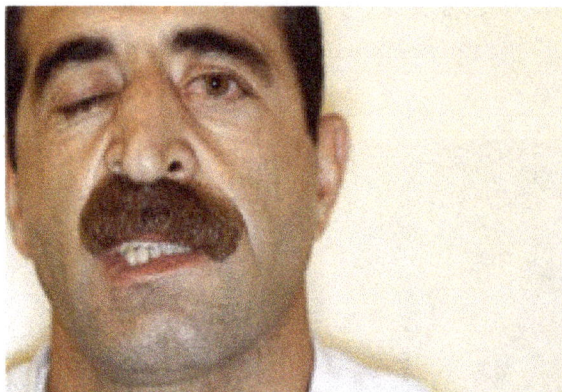

Figure 17. Four months after operation, minimal muscle function has returned; lagophthalmos will be addressed later.

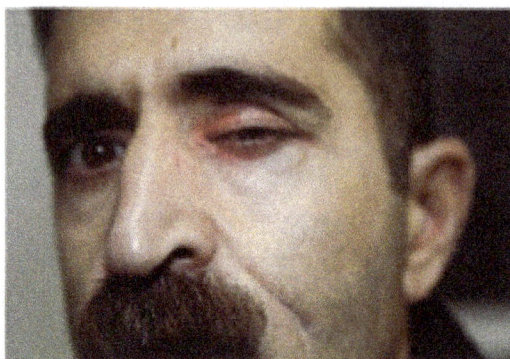

Figure 18. Tendon transfer for the eye with the face contour nearly normal.

One- or two-stage free vascularized muscle transfers are the best options for facial reanimation but they are lengthy operations and more sophisticated than the static slings. Interest in the temporalis muscle transfer has been renewed but the results are inferior to the muscle transfers [18] (**Figures 19** and **20**).

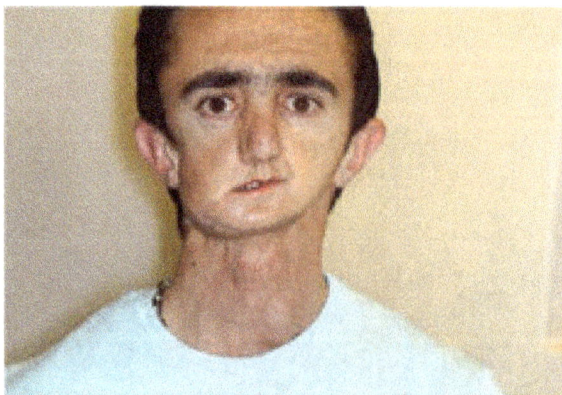

Figure 19. Facial palsy in a patient after reconstruction of the mandible due to childhood radiation-induced lower face atrophy.

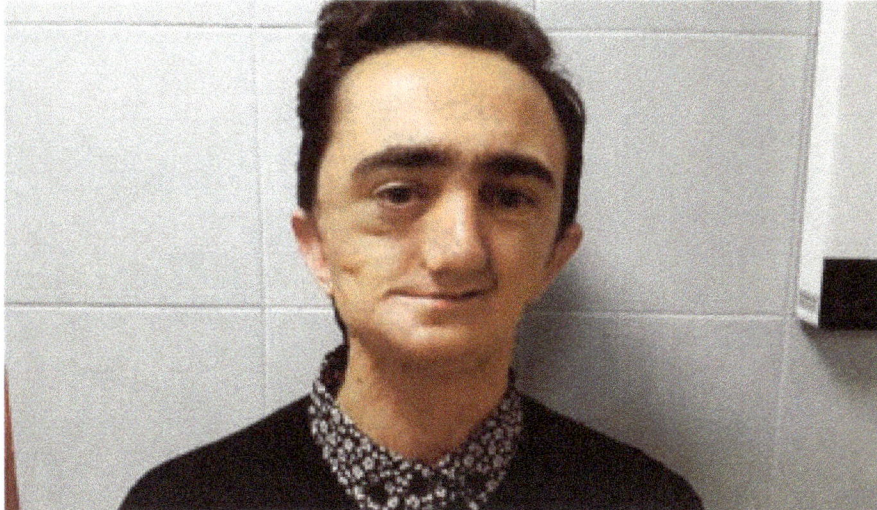

Figure 20. Temporalis transfer for right facial palsy.

The procedure of choice to regain involuntary smile is a two-stage transfer of the gracilis muscle. There are several candidate muscles in the literature, such as the pectoralis minor and latissimus dorsi (LD) as a one-stage muscle transfer (**Figure 21**).

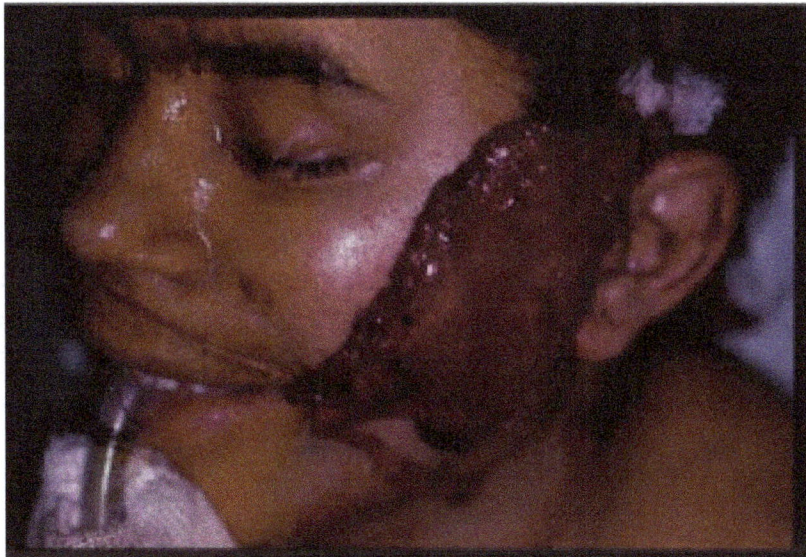

Figure 21. The one-stage LD muscle transfer, which can be done in one stage due to its long nerve.

At the first operation, a branch of the facial nerve on the healthy side is grafted and carried across by a sural nerve graft to the paralyzed side. The recommended route for nerve graft is across the face, through the upper lip and actually lying in the midface area, where at the second stage, a skin elevation is needed to insert the flap. Due to hazardous route of the cable graft, we think that a submental or frontal route is better suited for this operation because the nerve graft is safe when elevating the flaps at the second stage and also in future revision surgeries (**Figure 22**).

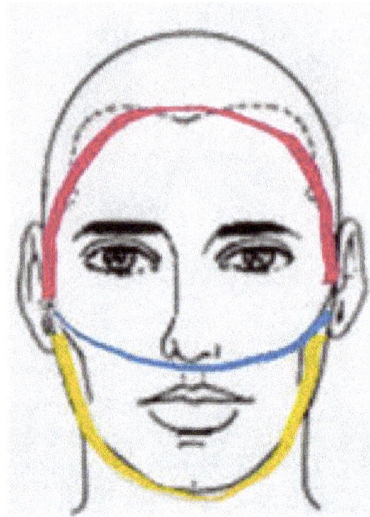

Figure 22. Blue is the recommended route; yellow and red routes are our preferred ways to transfer the nerve graft from one side of the face to the other side.

Six to nine months later, a segment of the gracilis muscle is transferred to the face and connected to the grafted nerve. The muscle becomes functional, providing movement on the paralyzed side. The gracilis transfer affords a better precision to the smile angle and greater movement of the commissure, when compared to temporalis transfer.

Terzis and Anesti used platysma muscle transfer to augment the function of or regulate the overactive previously transferred free vascularized muscle for oral sphincter control [19].

3.7.5.2. Synkinesis

Synkinesis is abnormal involuntary facial muscle movement during the voluntary movement of different muscle groups. For example, eye closure can result in simultaneous contraction of orbicularis oris or platysma contraction during smile. Other cranial nerves such as ocular and abducens have also synkinesis problems.

The problem seems to be the random growth or "miswiring" of facial nerve.

Management is a multimodality protocol which includes multiple session chemo-denervation with botulinium toxin and biofeedback facial muscle retraining and also surgical procedures such as small nerve graft or repair [20].

Choi et al. in a study of botulinum toxin injection in facial paralysis showed significant suppression of synkinesis and improvement of facial symmetry with resulting elevated quality of life, social interaction, personal appearance, and food intake [21].

Radiofrequency ablations are theoretically capable of reducing the injection sessions but are still in investigative stages. At present the best method of treatment for synkinesis is chemo-denervation with physical therapy [22–24].

3.8. Vestibulocochlear nerve

The vestibulocochlear nerve (eighth cranial nerve) is a pure sensory intracranial nerve (**Figure 23**). This nerve has two functions and hence two nerves: sound transmission and balance. The nerves originate from sensory receptors of internal ear to the brain stem and thence to the post-central gyrus and auditory cortex. The two most frequent etiologies of eighth nerve pathology are skull base trauma and vestibular schwannomas with the latter being the most common lesion.

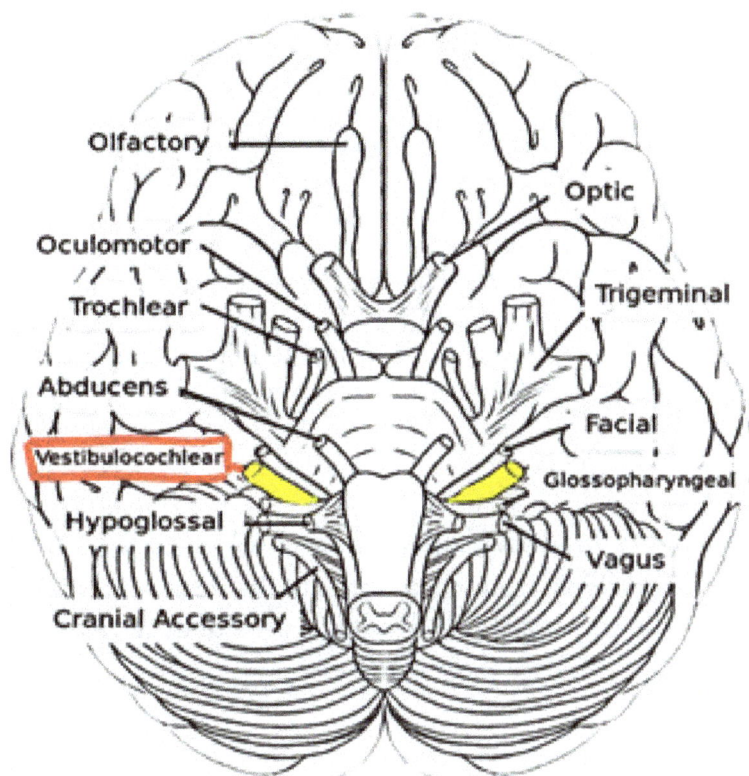

Figure 23. The eighth cranial nerve.

3.9. Glossopharyngeal

The ninth cranial nerve or glossopharyngeal nerve is a mixed nerve consisting of both sensory and motor nerve fibers (**Figure 24**). The origins of sensory fibers are pharynx, middle ear, posterior one-third of the tongue (including taste buds), and the carotid body and sinus. The motor fibers terminate at the parotid gland, the glands of the posterior tongue, and the stylopharyngeus muscle. Hwang et al. in a review article found that frequency of communication between the facial nerve and the vestibulocochlear nerve was the highest (82.3%) and the frequency of communication between the facial nerve and the glossopharyngeal nerve was the lowest (20%). Surgeons should be aware of the nerve communications, which are important during clinical examinations and surgical procedures of the facial nerves such as those communications involved in facial reconstructive surgery, neck dissection, and various nerve transfer procedures [25].

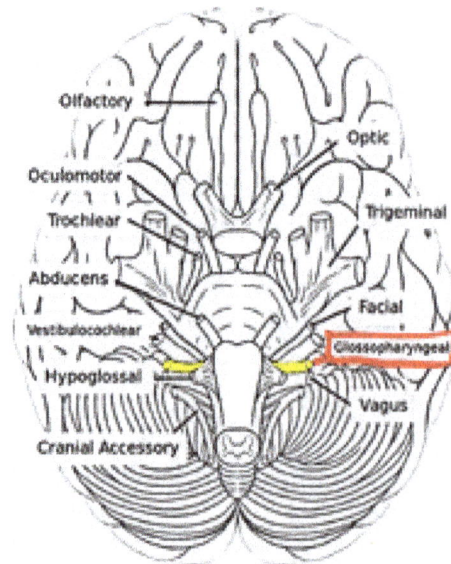

Figure 24. Ninth cranial nerve location at the undersurface of the brain.

The glossopharyngeal nerve is in danger of iatrogenic injury during tonsillectomy and the bilateral injury can be devastating [26].

3.10. Vagus nerve

The vagus nerve (**Figure 25**), from the Latin root meaning "wanderer," is the longest cranial nerve with far reaching functions, from vocal cords to the heart and finally the stomach and gallbladder. This nerve is at greatest risk in head and neck re-exploration.

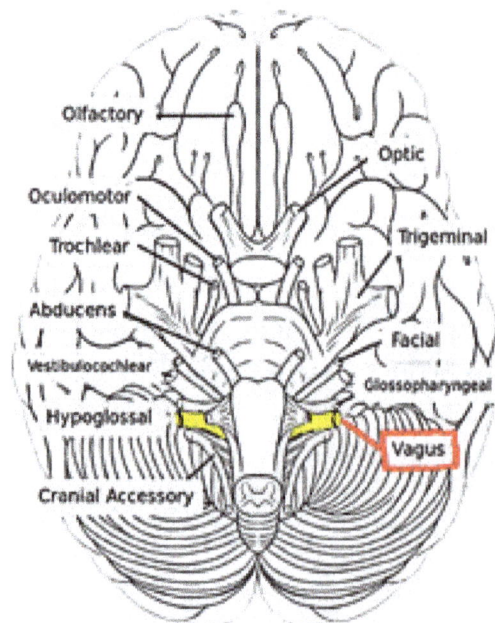

Figure 25. The 10th and the longest cranial nerve.

One of the important branches of the vagus nerve is RLN, the nightmare of head and neck surgery and especially thyroid surgery. Unrecognized RLN injury entails delayed phono-surgical intervention and laryngeal reinnervation.

Unilateral RLN damage is usually the complication of thyroid cancer surgery; in these instances when the nerve is involved in cancer, unilateral nerve resection or resection and nerve graft have been proposed [27].

Hong et al. [28] performed immediate direct anastomosis of RLNs injured during surgery for thyroid cancer; they found that patients undergoing immediate direct RLN anastomosis demonstrated better phonation and perceptually rated voice quality than those who did not undergo repair.

3.11. Spinal accessory nerve (SAN)

The accessory nerve is unique in that its name is based on a historical misunderstanding regarding its origin although it retains its original cranial nerve terminology; but contemporary nomenclature is more inclined toward spinal origin of this nerve, since the cranial part immediately joins the vagus nerve and the spinal part is considered the only and main part of the eleventh nerve [29] (**Figure 26**).

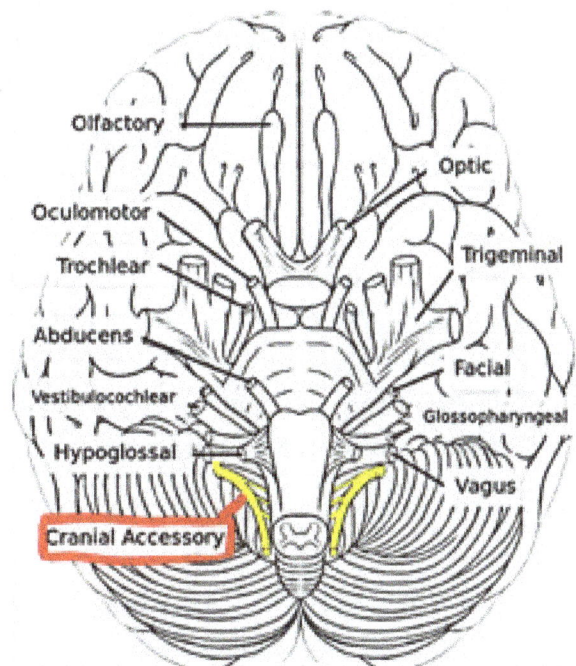

Figure 26. The 11th nerve; as the name implies, some authors think of this nerve as a spinal nerve.

During the past century, the anatomy and blood supply of SAN have been better understood (**Figure 27**). The importance of almost all of the SAN plexus to head, neck, and upper extremity motor and sensory functions has come to be realized. Because of this understanding, surgical neck dissection has become progressively more conservative toward preserving this nerve as much as possible.

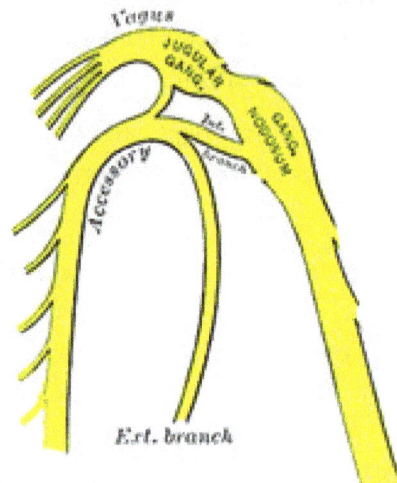

Figure 27. The relations of the SAN to vagus nerve (Gray's anatomy).

Iatrogenic injuries to the spinal accessory are not uncommon during lymph node biopsy of the posterior cervical triangle.

Park et al. review the operative techniques and surgical outcomes of 156 surgical repairs of the SAN following iatrogenic injury during lymph node biopsy procedures. SAN injuries present challenges for surgical exploration and repair because of the nerve's size and location in the Posterior cervical triangle. They concluded that patients with diminished or absent function achieved favorable functional outcomes by corrective surgery. Surgeons performing lymph node biopsy procedures in Zone I of posterior cervical triangle should be aware of the potential risk of injury to the SAN [30].

Nerve transfer between the SAN and the suprascapular nerve is a standard technique in brachial plexus surgery for shoulder reanimation. In cases of global brachial plexus injury, donor nerves are few and at times severely traumatized owing to extensive traction forces. Bhandari and Deb [31] offer the use of the contralateral SAN as an additional option in the reinnervation of an injured Suprascapular nerve in such circumstances.

3.12. Hypoglossal nerve

Use of the entire hypoglossal nerve for nerve transfer in obstetric palsy is not recommended because of major donor nerve morbidity in terms of feeding and speech problems (**Figure 28**).

The hypoglossal nerve to facial nerve transfer is one of the facial reanimation procedures, care must be taken to preserve the hypoglossal nerve for its primary function, and end-to-side nerve transfer is also mentioned in the literature. Beutner et al. have described the modified technique of the hypoglossal-facial-jump anastomosis without an interposition graft [32].

Al-thunyan et al. used a hemi-hypoglossal nerve transfer for biceps reinnervation in obstetric palsy in three infants with multiple root avulsions.

Elbow flexion was seen in two of the three operated patients with no reported feeding problem. Speech assessment was done at the 20–27 months of age and early speech development was unaffected [33].

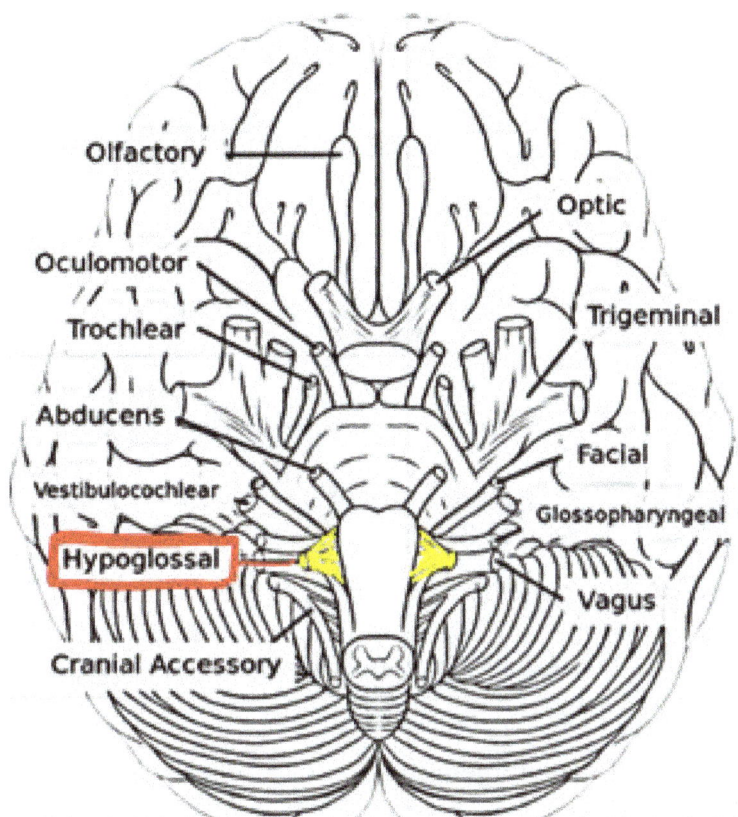

Figure 28. The 12th cranial nerve.

4. Summary

The knowledge of cranial nerves' anatomy is an important and integral part of head and neck surgery; we have discussed the cranial nerve anatomy and surgery, ablations, and reconstructions and several personal cranial nerve surgeries have been included in this chapter. The results indicate that patients are at greatest danger of cranial nerve damage during times of *stress* and that surgeons should take particular care to protect specific nerves in tough conditions.

Acknowledgements

We wish to thank all the patients who permitted us to show their faces.

Author details

Shahram Nazerani[1] and Tina Nazerani[2*]

*Address all correspondence to: tnazerani@yahoo.com

1 Rasool Akram General Hospital, Iran Medical University of Medical Sciences, Tehran, Iran

2 General Practitioner, Graz, Austria

References

[1] Clarke E, Jacyna LS. Nineteenth-century origins of neuroscientific concepts. Berkeley and Los Angeles: University of California Press. 1987.

[2] Shoja et al., 2007; Shaw, 1992.

[3] Flamm ES. Historical observations on the cranial nerves. J Neurosurg 1967;27:285–97 (Flamm, 1967; Shaw, 1992).

[4] Shaw JP. A history of the enumeration of the cranial nerves by European and British anatomists from the time of Galen to 1895, with comments on nomenclature. Clin Anat 1992;5.

[5] Davis MC, Griessenauer CJ, Bosmia AN, Tubbs RS, Shoja MM. The naming of the cranial nerves: a historical review. Clin Anat 2014;27:14–9

[6] Thiruvenkatarajan V, Van Wijk RM, Rajbhoj A. Cranial nerve injuries with supraglottic airway devices: a systematic review of published case reports and series. Anaesthesia 2015;70:344–59.

[7] Fokkema M, de Borst GJ, Nolan BW, Indes J, Buck DB, Lo RC, Moll FL, Schermerhorn ML, on behalf of the Vascular Study Group of New England. Clinical relevance of cranial nerve injury following carotid endarterectomy. Eur J Vasc Endovasc Surg 2014 Jan;47(1):2e7.

[8] van Riel D, Verdijk R, Kuiken T. The olfactory nerve: a shortcut for influenza and other viral diseases into the central nervous system. J Pathol 2015 Jan;235(2):277–87. doi: 10.1002/path.4461.

[9] Kumar R. Esthesioneuroblastoma: multimodal management and review of literature. World J Clin Cases 2015 Sep; 3(9):774–8. doi: 10.12998/wjcc.v3.i9.774 [published online Sep 16].

[10] Coelho DH, Costanzo RM. Posttraumatic olfactory dysfunction. Auris Nasus Larynx 2015 Oct. pii: S0385-8146(15)00200-X. doi: 10.1016/j.anl.2015.08.006 [Epub ahead of print].

[11] Sadagopan KA, Wasserman BN. Managing the patient with oculomotor nerve palsy. Curr Opin Ophthalmol 2013;24(5):438–47. doi: 10.1097/ICU.0b013e3283645a9b.

[12] Bagheri SC, Meyer RA, Khan HA, Kuhmichel A, Steed MB. Retrospective review of microsurgical repair of 222 lingual nerve injuries. J Oral Maxillofac Surg 2010;68(4):715–23. doi: 10.1016/j.joms.2009.09.111 [Epub 2009 Dec 29].

[13] Carr MM, Ross DA, Zuker RM. Cranial nerve defects incongenital facial palsy. J Otolaryngol 1997;26:80–7.

[14] Amer TA, El-Minawi HM, El-Shazly MI. Low-level versus high-level placement of gold plates in the upper eyelid in patients with facial palsy. Clin Ophthalmol 2011;5:891–5. doi: 10.2147/OPTH.S21491 [Epub 2011 June 30].

[15] Terzis JK, Karypidis D, Blink restoration in adult facial paralysis. Plast Reconstr Surg 2010;126(1):126–39.

[16] Rose EH. Autogenous fascia lata grafts: clinical applications in reanimation of the totally or partially paralyzed face. Plast Reconstr Surg 2005;116(1):20–32.

[17] Humphrey CD, McIff TE, Sykes KJ, et al. Suture biomechanics and static facial suspension. Arch Facial Plast Surg 2007;9(3):188–93.

[18] Byrne PJ, Kim M, Boahene K, et al. Temporalis tendon transfer as part of a comprehensive approach to facial reanimation. Arch Facial Plast Surg 2007;9(4):234–41.

[19] Terzis JK, Anesti K. Novel use of platysma for oral sphincter substitution or countering excessive pull of a free muscle. J Plast Reconstr Aesthet Surg 2013;66(8):1045–57. doi: 10.1016/j.bjps.2013.04.014 [Epub 2013 May 17].

[20] Terzis JK, Karypidis D. Therapeutic strategies in post-facial paralysis synkinesis in adult patients. Plast Reconstr Surg 2012;129(6):925e–939e. doi: 10.1097/PRS. 0b013e318230e758.

[21] Choi KH, Rho SH, Lee JM, Jeon JH, Park SY, Kim J. Botulinum toxin injection of both sides of the face to treat post-paralytic facial synkinesis. J Plast Reconstr Aesthet Surg 2013;66(8):1058–63.

[22] Mehta RP, Weknick Robinson M, Hadlock TA. Validation of the synkinesis assessment questionnaire. Laryngoscope 2007;117(5):923–6.

[23] Husseman J, Mehta RP. Management of synkinesis. Facial Plast Surg 2008;24(2):242–9.

[24] Vanswearingen J. Facial rehabilitation: a neuromuscular reeducation, patient-centered approach. Facial Plast Surg 2008;24(2):250–9.

[25] Hwang K, Song JS, Yang SC. Communications between the facial nerve and the vestibulocochlear nerve, the glossopharyngeal nerve, and the cervical plexus. J Craniofac Surg 2015 Oct;26(7):2190–2.

[26] Trinidade A, Philpott CM. Bilateral glossopharyngeal nerve palsy following tonsillectomy: a very rare and difficult complication of a common procedure. J Laryngol Otol 2015;129(4):392–4 [Epub 2015 Feb 20].

[27] Yumoto E, Sanuki T, Kumai Y. Immediate recurrent laryngeal nerve reconstruction and vocal outcome. Laryngoscope 2006;116:1657–61

[28] Hong JW, Roh TS, Yoo HS, Hong HJ, Choi HS, Chang HS, Park CS, Kim YS. Outcome with immediate direct anastomosis of recurrent laryngeal nerves injured during thyroidectomy. Laryngoscope 2014;124:1402–8.

[29] Ryan S, Blyth P, Duggan N, Wild M, Al-Ali S. Is the cranial accessory nerve really a portion of the accessory nerve? Anatomy of the cranial nerves in the jugular foramen. Anatomical Science International/Japanese Association of Anatomists 2007;82(1):1–7.

[30] Park SH, Esquenazi Y, Kline DG, Kim DH. Surgical outcomes of 156 spinal accessory nerve injuries caused by lymph node biopsy procedures. J Neurosurg Spine 2015;23(4): 518–25. doi: 10.3171/2014.12.SPINE14968. [Epub 2015 June 26]

[31] Bhandari PS, Deb P. Use of contralateral spinal accessory nerve for ipsilateral suprascapular neurotization in global brachial plexus injury: a new technique. J Neurosurg Spine 2016;24(1):186–8. doi: 10.3171/2015.4.SPINE15108 [Epub 2015 September 25].

[32] Beutner D, Luers JC, Grosheva M. Hypoglossal-facial-jump-anastomosis without an interposition nerve graft. Laryngoscope 2013;123(10):2392–6. doi: 10.1002/lary.24115 [Epub 2013 May 13].

[33] Al-Thunyan A, Al-Qattan MM, Al-Meshal O, Al-Husainan H, Al-Assaf A. Hemihypoglossal nerve transfer for obstetric brachial plexus palsy: report of 3 cases. J Hand Surg Am 2015;40(3):448–51. doi: 10.1016/j.jhsa.2014.11.018 [Epub 2015 January 21].

8

Complications of Orthognathic Surgery

Reza Tabrizi and Hassan Mir Mohammad Sadeghi

Abstract

Orthognathic surgery is a common approach for treatment of maxillofacial deformities. Sagittal split ramus osteotomy (SSRO) is one of the most common techniques used to treat various mandibular deformities. A LeFort I osteotomy is suggested in deformities of the maxilla and can be used along with SSRO or intra-oral vertical ramus osteotomy (IVRO).The aim of orthognathic surgery is to improve function and facial appearance; this benefits the patient psychologically and socially. Common complications which may occur in orthognathic surgery include vascular disease, temporomandibular joints (TMJ) problems, nerve damage, infection, bone necrosis, periodontal disease, vision impairment, hearing problems, hair loss, and neuropsychiatric problems. Rarely complications could be fatal. Because of the wide range of complications the surgeon should keep prevention protocols in mind and be prepared to treat them should they occur. In this chapter, common complications of various osteotomies in the mandible and maxilla are discussed.

Keywords: osteotomies, complications

1. Introduction

1.1. LeFort osteotomies

Midface osteotomies have been used to correct maxillary-zygomatic deformities, and historically have been classified anatomically based on the Guerin-LeFort fracture classification [1]. The first total LeFort I osteotomy was performed by Wassmund in 1927 for correction of the skeletal open bite [2]. In spite of all the advancements made in the field of orthognathic surgery, a variety of complications are documented [3]. These include maxillary sinusitis, loss of tooth vitality, sensory nerve morbidity, aseptic necrosis, vascular complications (i.e., arteriovenous fistulae or hemorrhage) nasal septum deviation, unfavorable fractures of the skull base and pterygoid plates, ophthalmic complications (including blindness) malpositioning, nonunion, maxilla instability, and relapse [4].

1.2. Hemorrhage

Excessive bleeding has been reported as a common complication of LeFort osteotomies. The incidence of life-threatening hemorrhage in maxillary osteotomies is reported in approximately 1% [5]. The descending palatine artery is the most common source for mild to moderate bleeding during LeFort I osteotomy and delayed bleeding afterward. The descending palatine artery damage may occur during the medial wall osteotomy. Injury to the descending palatine artery during LeFort I osteotomy can be minimized by limiting the osteotomy to 30 mm posterior to the piriform rim in females and to 35 mm in males[6]. In maxillary superior repositioning, bone removal around the descending palatine artery is a common cause of vascular injury. If the surgeon encounters the descending palatine artery, it should be cauterized. The internal maxillary artery is the most frequently cited source of massive hemorrhage [7]. Meticulous placement of the curved osteotome in the pterygomaxillary junction is important to avoid injury to the internal maxillary artery and its branches. Turvey and Fonseca reported that the main trunk of the maxillary artery was most vulnerable to the damage within the pterygopalatine fossa in the lateral position and they recommended angling the posterior lateral maxillary osteotomy downward to avoid damaging the artery [8]. Packing is suggested as the first attempt to tamponade the hemorrhage. In delayed bleeding after LeFort I osteotomy, the surgeon should reopen surgical site and move the maxilla downward to find the bleeding source (**Figure 1**). In many cases, direct visualization of the bleeding source and cauterization of injured vessels stops the hemorrhage (**Figure 2**). Several techniques have been suggested to control bleeding from the internal maxillary artery such as ligation of the external carotid artery and angiographic embolization. Emergency access to vascular embolization is crucial. If a patient has severe bleeding, the surgeon should not waste time and intervene immediately. The collateral arteries and the anastomoses between circulations lead to the limited success of surgical ligation of the external carotid artery [9]. A recent study recommended use of tranexamic acid irrigation in obviating perioperative blood loss during orthognathic surgery [10].

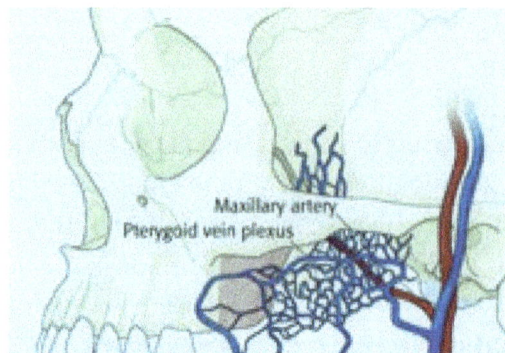

Figure 1. Possible bleeding sources during LeFort I osteotomy.

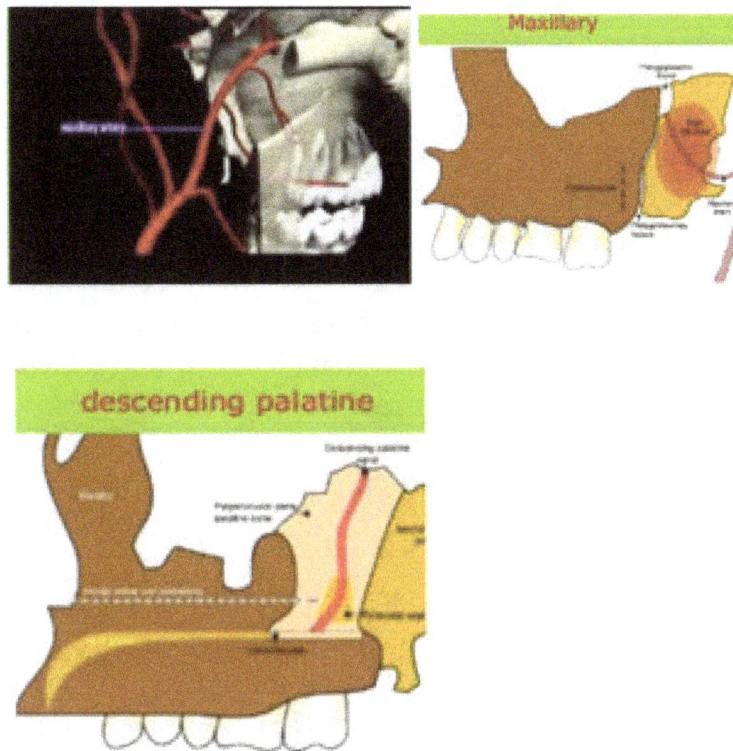

Figure 2. Relationship of osteotomy sites and major hemorrhage sources during LeFort I osteotomy.

1.3. Neurosensory deficit

The infraorbital nerve may be compressed, retracted or transected inadvertently during subperiosteal dissection.

Infraorbital nerve injury may have resulted from incorrect separation during disimpaction.

As are the cases with bilateral sagittal ramus osteotomy, nerve sensitivity may return within 6–12 months [11].

The absence of post-operatory sensitivity after a LeFort I procedure was documented in a study that applied both objective and subjective tests. The results showed a greater incidence of insensitivity in the region above the upper lip, followed by the lower lip and the chin, as was observed in bimaxillary procedures [12]. Neurosensory alterations are normally immediately perceived in the post-operatory period. They are the result of traction of the infraorbital nerve and direct trauma to the anterior, medial, and posterior superior alveolar nerves, as well as to the nasopalatine nerve and the descending palatal nerve [13]. A study performed at the University of North Carolina on patients undergoing bilateral Sagittal split ramus osteotomy (SSRO) reported that 98% of the patients presented altered sensitivity of the chin 1 month after the operation; with 81% of these patients still presenting with this alteration 6 months after the operation [14]. It is recommended that the patient be advised of possible neurosensory alterations in pre-operatory visits, thus reducing the patient's post-operatory anxiety [15]. Many studies confirm the return of neurosensory function up to 1 year after surgery [11].

1.4. Tooth sensitivity

An osteotomy closer than 5 mm of the apices of the teeth has risk of root injuries[16]. In superior repositioning of the maxilla by more than 6 mm, saving of 5 mm margin is not always possible because of the infraorbital foramen position [4]. After orthognathic surgery, loss of vascularity of the dentition is rare, but initial loss of response to pulpal stimulation is common. Long-term suppressed response to stimulation can occur, but does not necessarily mean a tooth requires endodontic therapy. Although some teeth may eventually become necrotic and require endodontic treatment, many teeth recover without treatment and return to normal coloration and respond to pulp testing [17]. De Jongh et al. studied electric and thermal pulp testing of 10 patients after LeFort I osteotomy in compared to 10 control patients without osteotomy. Their study showed that 71% of 128 teeth were responsive to electric and thermal pulp stimulation and 93% of 136 teeth in the controls [18].

1.5. Maxillary sinusitis

Sinusitis after LeFort I osteotomy is uncommon, with a reported incidence of septic complications of 0.5–4.8% [19]. Possible explanations for postoperative maxillary sinusitis following LeFort I osteotomy were pre-existing sinus disease or non-viable bone fragments left in the maxillary sinus (**Figure 3**) [20]. A recent study by Valestar et al. showed LeFort I procedure did not influence already existing physical or mental complaints, and nasal ventilation was not negatively affected. However, evaluation of sino-nasal pathology should be emphasized in the preoperative work-up [19]. A recent study by Nocini et al. suggested that LeFort I osteotomies can affect the maxillary sinus. The postoperative radiologic views of the maxillary sinus showed inflammation and rhinosinusitis symptoms after LeFort osteotomies. Larger long-term studies are warranted to clarify the postoperative outcomes and complications (**Figure 4**) [21].

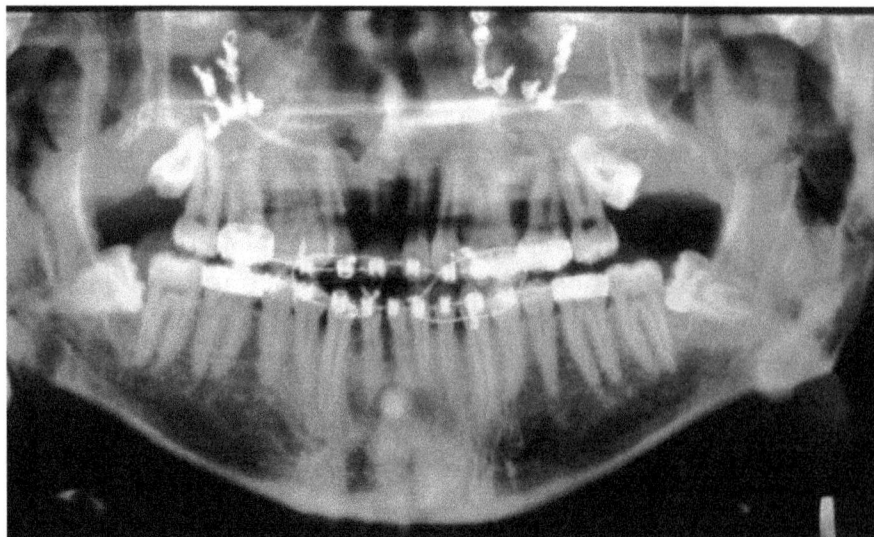

Figure 3. Maxillary sinusitis after LeFort I osteotomy.

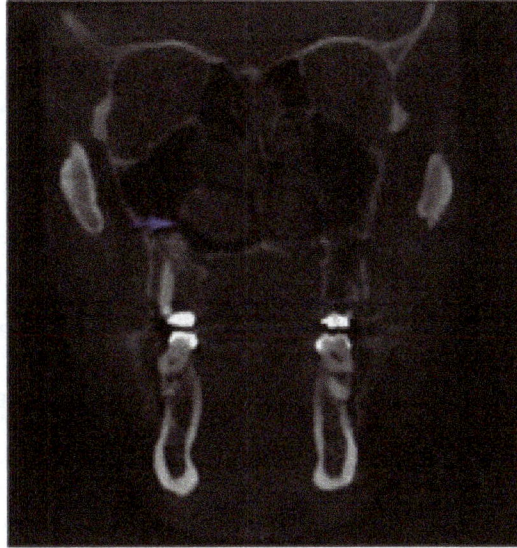

Figure 4. Radiologic findings: postoperative computed tomography scan displaying interruption of the medial walls [21].

1.6. Nose deformity

Septal malposition may occur during LeFort osteotomy and cause nasal deviation. A possible reason for a cartilagenous septum deviation after a maxillary osteotomy is dislocation by a partially deflated cuff during extubation. Manual inspection of the nares after extubation is important, yet often forgotten [22]. Nasal ventilation generally improves after orthognathic surgery [19]. The most common reason for postoperative nasal-septal deviation is compression or displacement from inadequate bone removal of the nasal crest of the maxilla or inadequate trimming of the cartilagenous septum (**Figure 5**) [9].

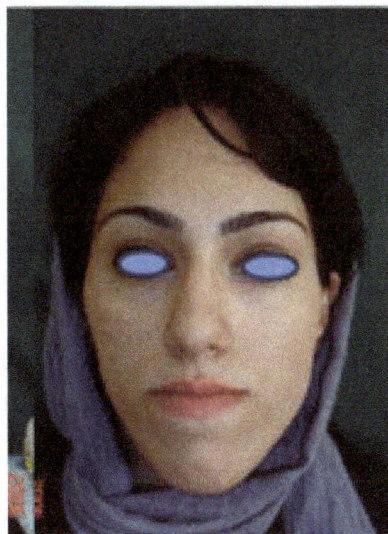

Figure 5. Severe nasal deviation after LeFort I osteotomy.

1.7. Aseptic necrosis

Avascular necrosis of the maxilla after LeFort I osteotomy has been reported [23]. Usually, these complications relate to the degree of vascular compromise and occur in less than 1% of cases. Rupture of the descending palatine artery during surgery, postoperative vascular thrombosis, perforation of palatal mucosa when splitting the maxilla into segments, or partial stripping of palatal soft tissues to increase maxillary expansion may impair blood supply to the maxillary segments. Sequelae of compromised vasculature include loss of tooth vitality, development of periodontal defects, tooth loss, or loss of major segments of alveolar bone or the entire maxilla (**Figure 6**) [24]. The risk is increased in patients with anatomical irregularities, such as craniofacial dysplasia's, orofacial clefts, or vascular anomalies [5]. The treatment of avascular necrosis of the maxilla is not easily manageable [25]. Regarding no treatment protocol has been established, aseptic necrosis of the maxilla should be treated by maintenance of optimal hygiene, antibiotic therapy to prevent secondary infection, heparinization, and hyperbaric oxygenation [24]. In such cases, it is evident that there is a serious problem with the tissue perfusion immediately postoperatively and the patient must be taken back to the theatre immediately to reposition the segment; delay only makes it worse [26].

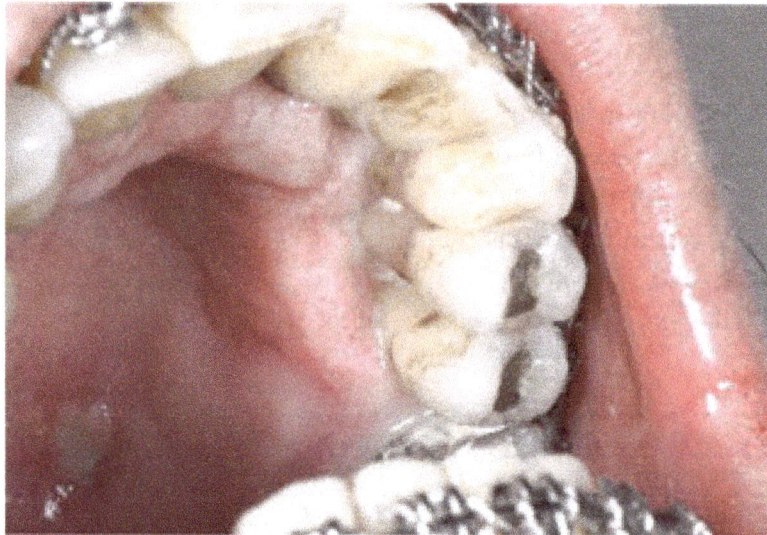

Figure 6. Initial aspect of the aseptic maxillary necrosis on the seventh postoperative day [24].

1.8. Unfavorable fractures

Unfavorable fractures may consist of pterygoid plate, sphenoid bone, and middle cranial fossa fractures. Lanigan and Guest demonstrated pterygomaxillary dysjunction using a curved osteotome and described high-level fractures of the pterygoid plates with disruption of the pterygopalatine fossa which could extend to the skull base [27]. Unfavorable pterygoid plate fracture is well studied and documented (**Figure 7**) [28]. Postoperative CT scans indicated that the prevalence of unfavorable fractures of the pterygomaxillary region may be more than previous expectations. Many of these unfavorable fractures are unobserved as there was no

CSF leak because of a local soft tissue seal [29]. Renicke et al. reported the incidence of pterygoid plate fracture was 58% following LeFort I osteotomy using postoperative CT scans [30].

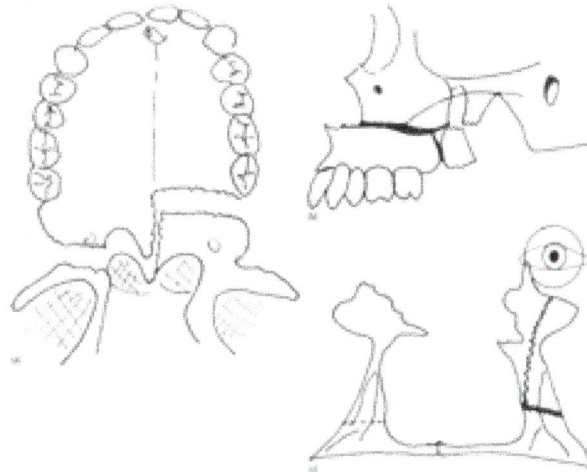

Figure 7. Possible lines of bad split during LeFort I osteotomy.

1.9. Improper maxillary repositioning

Several factors are responsible for improper maxillary repositioning such as missing a centric relation-centric occlusion discrepancy preoperatively; failure to achieve the desired maxillary position during isolated maxillary surgery, failure to seat the condyle because of inadequate removal of posterior bony interference and inaccurate vertical positioning [9]. Improper maxillary positioning may occur in correction of vertical maxillary excess. In a study by the first author, the incidence of under-correction (25%) was more than over-correction (7.5%)

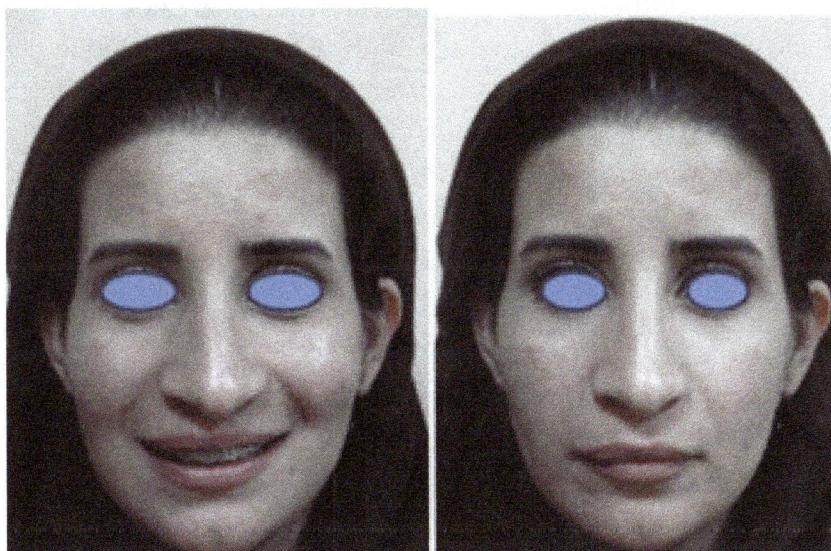

Figure 8. Over-correction after maxillary superior repositioning.

(**Figure 8**). Five millimeter was considered as a cutoff point for tooth shows at rest and 15 mm at the maximum smile. When tooth show at rest was more than 5 mm presurgically, 50.5% of clinical predictions did not follow the clinical results, and 75% of clinical predictions revealed the same results when the tooth show was less than 5 mm. When the amount of tooth shown in the maximum smile was more than 15 mm presurgically, 75% of clinical predictions did not follow clinical results, and 25% of the predictions met the same results in the maximum smile was less than. Clinical predictions based on the tooth show at rest and at the maximum smile did not have a reliable correlation with clinical results in maxillary superior repositioning. The risk of errors in predictions raised when the amount of superior repositioning of the maxilla increased. Generally, surgeons had a tendency to under-correct rather than over-correct. Also clinical prediction is used as a guideline by many surgeons, and it may be associated with variable clinical results [31].

1.10. Trigemino-cardiac reflex

Trigemino-cardiac reflex (TCR) is characterized by cardiac arrhythmia, ectopic beats, atrioventricular block, bradycardia, syncope, vomiting, and asystole. This life-threatening condition has been documented during simple zygomatic arch elevations, repositioning of blowout and maxillary fractures, orthognathic surgery, and nasoethmoidal fractures [32]. Besides evaluation of at-risk patients (e.g., children and patients with a medical history of cardiac disease) and high-risk surgeries (e.g., strabismus), some authors suggested using ketamine for anesthetic induction to decrease the oculocardiac reflex in children undergoing strabismus surgery [32]. Predisposing factors besides cardiac disease are hypoxia and hypercarbia, and use of opioids and β-blockers. TCR has been identified with a sudden onset of parasympathetic hypotension, apnea, or gastric hypermotility during stimulation of any of the sensory branches of the trigeminal nerve. In some cases, stopping the surgery has resulted in recovery of a normal rhythm; in other cases, anticholinergic drugs and cardiac massage have been mentioned. It is recommended that the anesthesiology team be informed that they may be prepared for mobilization in case of adverse effects. In every high-risk case presented in the classification, prophylactic administration of, for example, 0.5 mg atropine IV, right before any surgical manipulation known to be risky for TCR is mandatory [32].

1.11. Ophthalmic complications

Potential ophthalmic complications following LeFort I osteotomy includes decrease in visual acuity, extraocular muscle dysfunction, neuroparalytic keratitis, and lacrimal apparatus problems including epiphora [33]. Visual impairment after LeFort I osteotomy may be due to inappropriate separation of the pterygomaxillary junction and resulting fractures extending to the pterygoid plates, sphenoid bone, orbital floor, optic canal, or the skull base. It may damage the optic nerve or its vascular supply. Hemorrhage from the descending palatine artery or sphenopalatine artery in LeFort I osteotomy may be considered as a reason for systemic hypotension. Hemorrhage from the pterygopalatine fossa may leak the orbital cavity through the inferior orbital fissure and increase intraocular pressure (IOP). Hypotensive anesthesia is useful during a maxillofacial operation for blood loss control and enhancing the visibility in the surgical field. The blood flow to the globes may be changed by elevated IOP or dropped systemic blood pressure. Hypotensive anesthesia may potentially reduce the blood supply to the retina and choroid and may cause embolism of the vessels or infarction of the optic nerve. The effect of hypotensive anesthesia on visual impairment has not been clarified yet [34].

1.12. Nasolacrimal duct obstruction

Nasolacrimal duct obstruction (NLDO) after maxillary orthognathic surgery is rare. The absence of an NLDO after LeFort I osteotomy is reasonable because the distance from the nasal opening of the NLD to the levels of osteotomy should be at least 5 mm. The normal distance between the NLD nasal opening and the nasal floor is 11–17 mm. LeFort I osteotomy should be performed 5 mm above the nasal floor. The distal to the proximal part of the NLD is vulnerable to be obstructed after maxillary osteotomy. Secondary inflammatory changes associated with an indirect injury of the NLD lead to obstruction. So surgeons should be aware of the risk of NLDO after orthognathic surgery (**Figures 9–11**); this can be managed by dacryocystorhinostomy with high success rate [35].

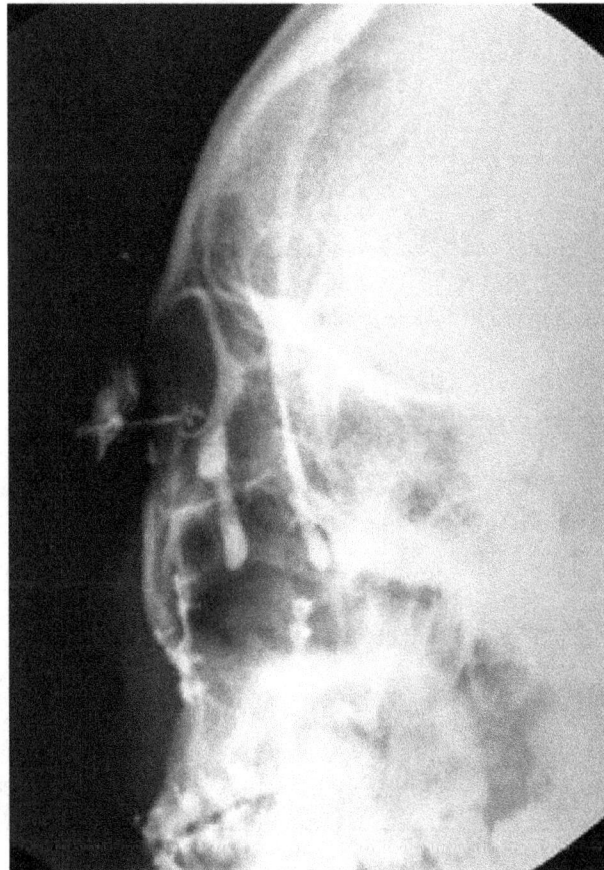

Figure 9. Representative dacryocystograms showing obstruction of the nasolacrimal duct in a patient who underwent orthognathic surgery and complained of permanent epiphora [35].

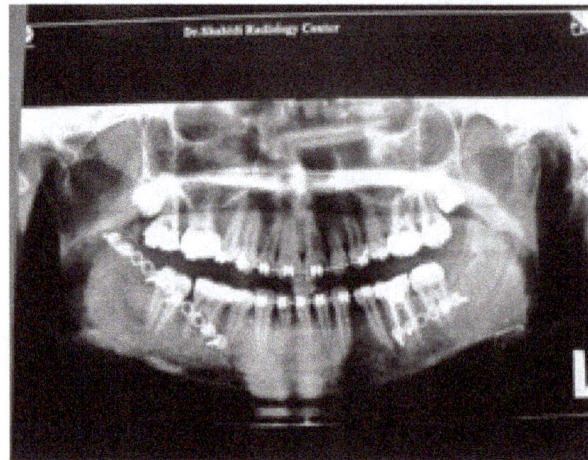

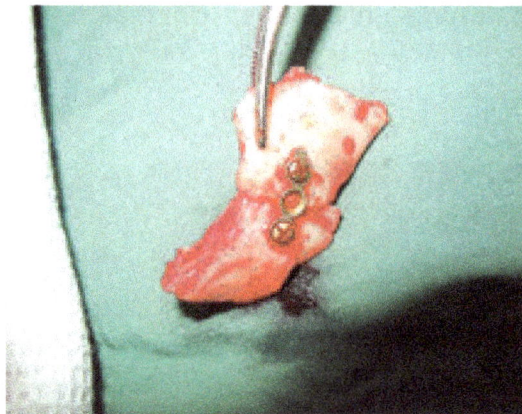

Figure 10. (A) Bad split occurred on the right side. (B) Fixation of bone fragment was done and replaced.

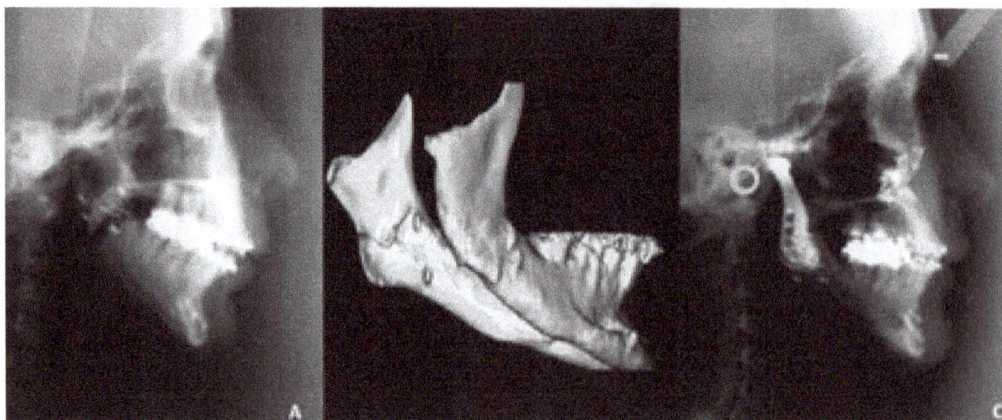

Figure 11. Complete destruction of condyle in a patient, who had undergone orthognathic surgery, was re-treated with the aid of temporomandibular joint prostheses. Before surgery (A), 3D image of the mandible showing bilateral absence of condyles (B), and after surgery (C) [53].

1.13. Nonunion of segments

Nonunion of segments in conventional LeFort I osteotomy is rare. In segmental osteotomy the risk of nonunion is higher. A good vascular pedicle and bone grafts are crucial. Additional stability of the maxillary segments after fixation with miniplates was suggested by the use of palatal dressing plates. Use of split with intermaxillary fixation may be useful. Three-dimensional fixation or immobilization can therefore be gained by using miniplates superiorly on the bony aspect, a dressing plate on the palatal aspect, and a wired-in final surgical wafer on the occlusal aspect of the dentoalveolar segments [36]. If nonunion occurs the surgical site should be reopened, fibrous tissue removed and proper rigid fixation be used for predictable union of segments.

1.14. Tooth damage

Tooth damage in segmental osteotomy is not uncommon. In LeFort I, the risk of damage to the teeth roots increases when the horizontal osteotomy line is 5 mm or less. Close proximity to interdental osteotomy cuts or to screws may cause tooth damage, and pulp necrosis [36]. The pulpal blood flow of teeth adjacent to vertical osteotomies of LeFort I segmental maxillary osteotomies has been reported to be decreased significantly at 4 days after surgeries for lateral incisors, canines, and premolars. However, recovery was seen 56 days after operations. The central incisors and teeth that are distant from the vertical osteotomy have blood flow without significant change [37]. It is advocated that presurgical orthodontic separation of the roots by at least 2 mm at the cementoenamel junction and 4 mm at the apical third be maintained to avoid vascular compromise or damage to the roots adjacent to interdental osteotomies [36].

2. Sagittal split osteotomy

Sagittal split osteotomy (SSO) is a conventional technique to correct mandibular excess or retrognathia. Since its introduction by Trauner and Obwegeser, SSO has undergone numerous modifications and improvements [38].

2.1. Neurosensory disturbance

In SSO, the inferior alveolar nerve (IAN) may be injured and cause neurosensory disturbance (NSD) in the lower lip. The NSD caused by damage to the IAN is reportedly 9–84.6% [39, 40]. Even with careful surgery, injury to the IAN appears unpredictable. Multiple factors are considered responsible for the development of NSD after SSO, including fixation methods, patient age and surgical procedures, improper splinting, magnitude of mandibular movement, experience of the surgeon, and timing of the postoperative neurosensory evaluation [40]. Injury to the IAN may happen with direct and indirect intraoperative trauma and results in change of sensibility or altered sensation of the lower lip and/or mental region. It may lead the negative effect on patients' normal functions such as eating, drinking, speech, and social interaction. NSD may affect patients' everyday lives and can have social or psychological problems [41].

The position of the canal is important in NSD following SSO because the canal position is impacted by osteotomy design and fixation techniques. Nowadays, technologies and software help to evaluate the canal by using CBCT data. An increased distance between the canal and cortical bone presurgically decreased the incidence of postoperative NSD, and high bone density increased of the risk of postoperative NSD. A short post-operation assessment comparing monocortical and bicortical fixation in a monkey model, showed that IAN function was better with plate fixation than screw fixation [42].

2.2. Unfavorable split

An unfavorable fracture, called a "bad split" although infrequent in the hands of an experienced operator, occasionally develop and can lead to intraoperative difficulties as well as postoperative relapse [43]. Frequently cited reasons for bad split include incomplete osteotomies, using osteotomes that are too large, attempting to split the segments too rapidly presence of impacted third molars, misdirecting the medial osteotomy upward toward the condyle and placement of the medial osteotomy too far superior to the lingula [44].

Synonyms used for bad split include "buccal cortical plate fracture" (proximal segment) and "lingual cortical plate fracture" (distal segment) [45]. A bad split can occur during SSO of the mandible regarding precautions. The incidence of bad split is low (0.7% of all SSOs) and patients sometimes have uneventful healing. A significant decrease in incidence did not report during the 20-year period, and neither technical progress nor the surgeon's experience further decreased the frequency of bad splits [45]. It was reported that older patients experienced more bad splits than younger patients [46]. The length of the medial osteotomy line—short or long —did not alter the prevalence of a bad split. The bone thickness of the ramus may affect the type of fracture pattern on the medial side of the ramus [47]. It is clear that certain mandibular anatomic differences can increase the risk of a bad split during SSO [44]. Use of splitters and separators instead of chisels does not increase the risk of a bad split and is therefore safe with predictable results [48].

2.3. Infection

Postoperative infection was reported in studies of patients undergoing bilateral sagittal ramus osteotomy in a period ranging from 5 days to up to a year after surgery. Infections required antibiotic therapy, and in some cases, the patients underwent surgical drainage. osteomyelitis in bilateral sagittal ramus osteotomy was reported [11]. The rate of infection after SSO is up to 11.3%. Infection after SSO is within normal range for a clean-contaminated procedure. Rigid fixation of the osteotomy may decrease the need for hardware removal [49].

2.4. Excessive bleeding

In the literature, there were no uniform criteria defining bleeding complications. Incidence varied between 0.39 and 38% ranging from slight to a life-threatening hemorrhage.

Minor bleeding in SSOs can usually be easily managed by using local anesthetics containing 1:100,000 adrenalines injected before the operation, electrocautery or compression. Excessive blood loss may due to surgical injury of larger vessels. It was reported that excessive blood loss happen mainly to maxillary surgery and the need for blood transfusion in mandibular operations is rarely necessary [50].

2.5. Condylar resorption

Condylar resorption (CR) or condylysis can be defined as progressive change of condylar shape with a reduction in mass. Most patients have a decrease in posterior face height, retrognathism, and progressive anterior open bite with clockwise rotation of the mandible. CR may be defined as osteoarthrosis and can be categorized as primary (idiopathic) and secondary. Current evidence on CR is not clear but seen more in female with mandibular deficiency and high mandibular plane angle after bimaxillary surgery; a change in occlusal plane (counterclockwise rotation) may be associated with condylar resorption after orthognathic surgery [51]. It was hypothesized that condylar remodeling is due to an imbalance between mechanical stress applied to the temporomandibular joints (TMJ) and patient' adaptive capacities. It mainly occurs in 14 to 50-years-old women with pre-existing TMJ dysfunction, estrogen deficiency, and class II malocclusion with a high mandibular plane angle, a diminished posterior facial height and posteriorly inclined condylar neck. Mandibular advancement superior to 10 mm, counterclockwise rotation of the mandible, and posterior condylar repositioning were associated with an increased risk of CROS. Treatment consists of reoperation in case of degradation after an inactivity period of at least 6 months [52].

2.6. Temporomandibular dysfunction

The effect of orthognathic surgeries on temporomandibular dysfunction(TMD) is controversial. Some studies support degrees of improvement of TMD [5, 54]. Patients with preexisting TMJ dysfunction undergoing orthognathic surgery, particularly mandibular advancement, are likely to have significant worsening of the TMJ dysfunction postsurgery. TMJ dysfunction must be closely evaluated, treated if necessary and monitored in the orthognathic surgery patients [55]. Use of lag screws, improper control of the proximal segments, and advancement more than 10 mm increases the risk of post-orthognathic TMD. Orthognathic surgery should not be used solely for management of TMD; patients having orthognathic treatment for correction of their dentofacial deformities with TMD problem had more improvement in their signs and symptoms than deterioration [56].

2.7. Postoperative airway problem

It is clear that mandibular set back can affect upper airway patency [57]. The amount of narrowing of the pharyngeal airway is smaller in patients undergoing bimaxillary surgery than in patients undergoing mandibular setback surgery [58]. Bimaxillary orthognathic surgery for correction of Class III malocclusion caused an increase of the total airway volume and improvement of polysomnography parameters [59]. Bimaxillary surgery rather than mandibular setback surgery should be used to correct a class III deformity and reduce the risk of obstructive sleep apnea; in fact, bimaxillary surgery may have less effect on the pharyngeal airway patency than mandibular setback surgery alone [60]. A recent study suggested that

BSSO presents less change in the pharyngeal airway space after mandibular setback surgery compared to intraoral vertical ramus osteotomy. Furthermore, bimaxillary surgery is superior to mandibular setback surgery alone for the correction of the prognathic mandible, particularly in patients with factors predisposing them to the development of breathing problems [61].

3. Intraoral vertical ramus osteotomy

Intraoral vertical ramus osteotomy (IVRO) is another approach for the correction of mandibular prognathism. It is very simple and rapid. The inherent anatomic architecture of the mandible poses little interference on the cut surface of the IVRO osteotomy site during mandibular setback, even in cases of severe asymmetry. In addition, because the segments are not fixed, no stress occurs while the distal segment is positioned with the condylar head during and after the osteotomy procedure. Moreover, IVRO has less chance of nerve damage during the osteotomy procedure than SSRO. In addition to advantages provided during the operation, this procedure has various postoperative advantages. It seems to have curable effects on most patients with preoperative TMD [9].

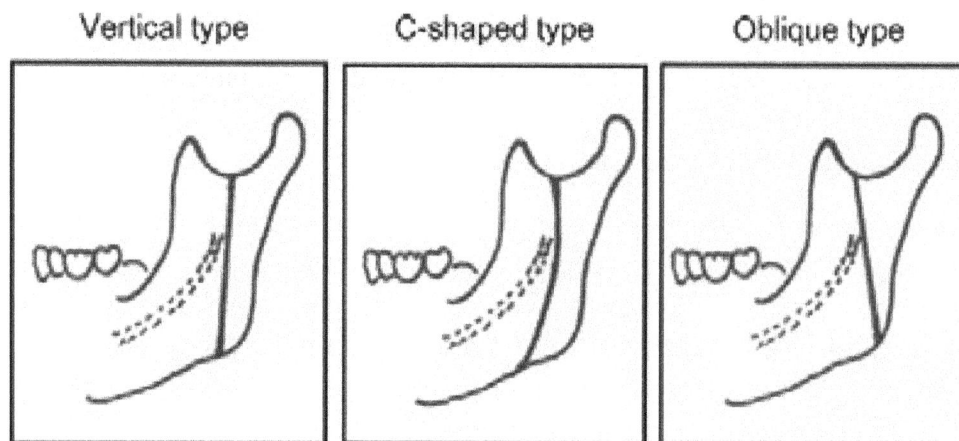

Figure 12. Classification of the shape of the osteotomy line [62].

During IVRO, inferior alveolar nerve (IAN) damage may occur due to the proximity of the vertical osteotomy to the IAN. Preoperatively, the surgeon should evaluate the lingula on radiographic views. The antilingular eminence on the lateral surface of the ramus should be detected. This small protuberance is located at the posterior one third from the posterior border of the ramus and about 10 mm above the occlusal plane of the lower molars in the vertical aspect, which corresponds to the opposite side of the mandibular foramen. The cut should begin 6–7 mm from the posterior border of the ramus. Kawase-Koga et al. classified the osteotomy line into three types, namely vertical, C-shaped, and oblique. The most complications occurred in the vertical type cases, and no complications were found in oblique type cases. Condylar luxation was found mainly in unilateral IVRO cases, and bony interference was found in bilateral IVRO cases. These results suggest that the oblique type of osteotomy line has the advantage of avoiding complications (**Figure 12**) [62].

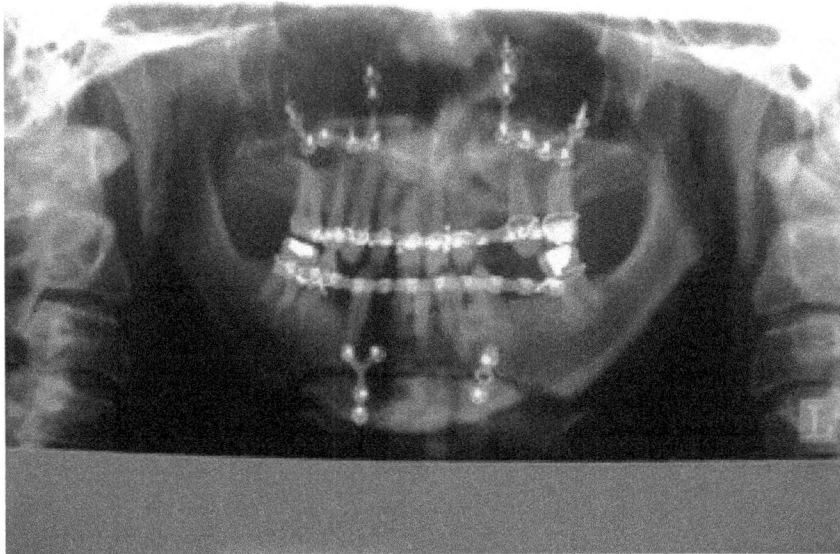

Figure 13. Condylar sagging at the (left side) after IVRO.

Condylar luxation and bony interference are major complications of IVRO [62]. The most troublesome sequelae are skeletal instability and antero-inferior condylar displacement (sag), with resultant unpredictability of postoperative mandibular position [63]. Condylar luxation is considered to be related to condylar sag, which occurs with the antero-inferior postoperative displacement of the proximal segment [62]. When the attachments of the masseter and medial pterygoid muscles to the proximal segment are removed extensively, large condylar sag occurs as a complication of IVRO. Condylar luxation is also related to forward force on the condyle from the lateral pterygoid muscle. Normally, the condyle is located in the anterior and inferior position within the glenoid fossa immediately after IVRO. It is gradually reseated into the original position after surgery with the application of intermaxillary elastics [64]. Several techniques have been reported to avoid condylar luxation and interference of the proximal segment. Suturing the periosteum of the segments around the incision with3–0 Vicryl to prevent sagging against the mandibular fossa has been suggested [64]. Rigid fixation is not recommended in IVRO and increases risk of post-operation open bite. Elastic therapy after osteotomy effectively decreases open bite due to the muscle tension (**Figure 13**).

Author details

Reza Tabrizi* and Hassan Mir Mohammad Sadeghi

*Address all correspondence to: tabmed@gmail.com

Department of Oral and Maxillofacial Surgery, Shahid Beheshti University of Medical Sciences, Tehran, Iran

References

[1] Kim, S.-G., and S.-S. Park, *Incidence of complications and problems related to orthognathic surgery*. Journal of Oral and Maxillofacial Surgery, 2007. 65(12): p. 2438–2444.

[2] Tabrizi, R., H. Pakshir, and B. Nasehi, *Does the type of maxillomandibular deformity influence complication rate in orthognathic surgery?* Journal of Craniofacial Surgery, 2015. 26(7): p. e643–e647.

[3] Wassmund, M., Leipzig: H. Meußer *Lehrbuch der praktischen Chirurgie des Mundes und der Kiefer*. Vol. 1. 1935: H. Meusser.

[4] Garg, S., and S. Kaur, *Evaluation of post-operative complication rate of Le Fort I osteotomy: a retrospective and prospective study*. Journal of Maxillofacial and Oral Surgery, 2014. 13(2): p. 120–127.

[5] Kramer, F.J., et al., *Intra- and perioperative complications of the LeFort I osteotomy: a prospective evaluation of 1000 patients*. Journal of Craniofacial Surgery, 2004. 15(6): p. 971–977; discussion 978–979.

[6] Li, K.K., J.G. Meara, and A. Alexander, Jr., Location of the descending palatine artery in relation to the Le Fort I osteotomy. Journal of Oral and Maxillofacial Surgery, 1996. 54(7): p. 822–825; discussion 826–827.

[7] Khanna, S., and A.B. Dagum, *A critical review of the literature and an evidence-based approach for life-threatening hemorrhage in maxillofacial surgery*. Annals of Plastic Surgery, 2012. 69(4): p. 474–478.

[8] Turvey, T., and R. Fonseca, *The anatomy of the internal maxillary artery in the pterygopalatine fossa: its relationship to maxillary surgery*. Journal of Oral Surgery (American Dental Association: 1965), 1980. 38(2): p. 92.

[9] Felice O'Rayan, A.S., *Complications with Orthognathic Surgery*, in *Oral and maxillofacial surgery*, M. Fonseca, Turvey, Editor. 2009, Saunders Elsevier. p. 419–489.

[10] Eftekharian, H., et al., *Effect of tranexamic acid irrigation on perioperative blood loss during orthognathic surgery: a double-blind, randomized controlled clinical trial*. Journal of Oral Maxillofacial Surgery, 2015. 73(1): p. 129–133.

[11] Sousa, C.S., and R.N.T. Turrini, *Complications in orthognathic surgery: a comprehensive review*. Journal of Oral and Maxillofacial Surgery, Medicine, and Pathology, 2012. 24(2): p. 67–74.

[12] Essick, G., et al., *Short-term sensory impairment after orthognathic surgery*. Oral and Maxillofacial Surgery Clinics of North America, 2001. 13(2): p. 295–314.

[13] Hummes, B., et al., *Complicações no tratamento cirúrgico da deficiência transversa do osso maxilar*. Stomatos, 2008. 14(27):p. 63–73.

[14] Essick, G.K., et al., *Facial altered sensation and sensory impairment after orthognathic surgery.* International Journal of Oral and Maxillofacial Surgery, 2007. 36(7): p. 577–582.

[15] Panula, K., K. Finne, and K. Oikarinen, *Incidence of complications and problems related to orthognathic surgery: a review of 655 patients.* Journal of Oral and Maxillofacial Surgery, 2001. 59(10): p. 1128–1136.

[16] Kahnberg, K., and H. Engström, *Recovery of maxillary sinus and tooth sensibility after Le Fort I osteotomy.* British Journal of Oral and Maxillofacial Surgery, 1987. 25(1): p. 68–73.

[17] Robl, M.T., B.B. Farrell, and M.R. Tucker, *Complications in orthognathic surgery: a report of 1000 cases.* Oral and Maxillofacial Surgery Clinics of North America, 2014. 26(4): p. 599–609.

[18] de Jongh, M., D. Barnard, and D. Birnie, *Sensory nerve morbidity following Le Fort I osteotomy.* Journal of Maxillofacial Surgery, 1986. 14: p. 10–13.

[19] Valstar, M.H., et al., *Maxillary sinus recovery and nasal ventilation after Le Fort I osteotomy: a prospective clinical, endoscopic, functional and radiographic evaluation.* International Journal of Oral Maxillofacial Surgery, 2013. 42(11): p. 1431–1436.

[20] Bell, C.S., W.J. Thrash, and M.K. Zysset, *Incidence of maxillary sinusitis following Le Fort I maxillary osteotomy.* Journal of Oral and Maxillofacial Surgery, 1986. 44(2): p. 100–103.

[21] Nocini, P.F., et al., *Is Le Fort I osteotomy associated with maxillary sinusitis?* Journal of Oral and Maxillofacial Surgery, 2016. 74(2): p. 400. e1–400. e12.

[22] Acebal-Bianco, F., et al., *Perioperative complications in corrective facial orthopedic surgery: a 5-year retrospective study.* Journal of Oral and Maxillofacial Surgery, 2000. 58(7): p. 754–760.

[23] Lanigan, D.T., J.H. Hey, and R.A. West, *Aseptic necrosis following maxillary osteotomies: report of 36 cases.* Journal of Oral and Maxillofacial Surgery, 1990. 48(2): p. 142–156.

[24] Pereira, F.L., et al., *Maxillary aseptic necrosis after Le Fort I osteotomy: a case report and literature review.* Journal of Oral and Maxillofacial Surgery, 2010. 68(6): p. 1402–1407.

[25] Kahnberg, K.E., and C. Hagberg, *The approach to dentofacial skeletal deformities using a multisegmentation technique.* Clinics in Plastic Surgery, 2007. 34(3): p. 477–484.

[26] Singh, J., et al., *Reconstruction of post-orthognathic aseptic necrosis of the maxilla.* British Journal of Oral Maxillofacial Surgery, 2008. 46(5): p. 408–410.

[27] Lanigan, D.T., and P. Guest, *Alternative approaches to pterygomaxillary separation.* International Journal of Oral Maxillofacial Surgery, 1993. 22(3): p. 131–138.

[28] Precious, D.S., et al., *Pterygoid plate fracture in Le Fort I osteotomy with and without pterygoid chisel: a computed tomography scan evaluation of 58 patients.* Journal of Oral Maxillofacial Surgery, 1993. 51(2): p. 151–153.

[29] Bhaskaran, A., et al., *A complication of Le Fort I osteotomy*. International Journal of Oral and Maxillofacial Surgery, 2010. 39(3): p. 292–294.

[30] Renick, B.M., and J.M. Symington, *Postoperative computed tomography study of pterygo-maxillary separation during the Le Fort I osteotomy*. Journal of Oral Maxillofacial Surgery, 1991. 49(10): p. 1061–1065; discussion 1065–1066.

[31] Tabrizi, R., B. Zamiri, and H. Kazemi, *Correlation of clinical predictions and surgical results in maxillary superior repositioning*. Journal of Craniofacial Surgery, 2014. 25(3): p. e220–e223.

[32] Lübbers, H.-T., et al., *Classification of potential risk factors for trigeminocardiac reflex in craniomaxillofacial surgery*. Journal of Oral and Maxillofacial Surgery, 2010. 68(6): p. 1317–1321.

[33] Lanigan, D.T., K. Romanchuk, and C.K. Olson, *Ophthalmic complications associated with orthognathic surgery*. Journal of Oral and Maxillofacial Surgery, 1993. 51(5): p. 480–494.

[34] Cheng, H.C., et al., *Blindness and basal ganglia hypoxia as a complication of Le Fort I osteotomy attributable to hypoplasia of the internal carotid artery: a case report*. Oral Surgery, Oral Medicine, Oral Pathology, Oral Radiology and Endodontology, 2007. 104(1): p. e27–e33.

[35] Jang, S.Y., et al., *Nasolacrimal duct obstruction after maxillary orthognathic surgery*. Journal of Oral and Maxillofacial Surgery, 2013. 71(6): p. 1085–1098.

[36] Ho, M., et al., *Surgical complications of segmental Le Fort I osteotomy*. British Journal of Oral and Maxillofacial Surgery, 2011. 49(7): p. 562–566.

[37] Emshoff, R., et al., *Effect of segmental Le Fort I osteotomy on maxillary tooth type-related pulpal blood-flow characteristics*. Oral Surgery, Oral Medicine, Oral Pathology, Oral Radiology and Endodontology, 2000. 89(6): p. 749–752.

[38] Trauner, R., and H. Obwegeser, *The surgical correction of mandibular prognathism and retrognathia with consideration of genioplasty. I. Surgical procedures to correct mandibular prognathism and reshaping of the chin*. Oral Surgery, Oral Medicine, Oral Pathology, 1957. 10(7): p. 677–689; contd.

[39] Al-Bishri, A., et al., *Neurosensory disturbance after sagittal split and intraoral vertical ramus osteotomy: as reported in questionnaires and patients' records*. International Journal of Oral and Maxillofacial Surgery, 2005. 34(3): p. 247–251.

[40] Kuroyanagi, N., et al., *Prediction of neurosensory alterations after sagittal split ramus osteotomy*. International Journal of Oral and Maxillofacial Surgery, 2013. 42(7): p. 814–822.

[41] Bruckmoser, E., et al., *Factors influencing neurosensory disturbance after bilateral sagittal split osteotomy: retrospective analysis after 6 and 12 months*. Oral Surgery, Oral Medicine, Oral Pathology and Oral Radiology, 2013. 115(4): p. 473–482.

[42] Rich, J., B.A. Golden, and C. Phillips, *Systematic review of preoperative mandibular canal position as it relates to postoperative neurosensory disturbance following the sagittal split ramus osteotomy.* International Journal of Oral and Maxillofacial Surgery, 2014. 43(9): p. 1076–1081.

[43] Smith, B.R., et al., *Mandibular ramus anatomy as it relates to the medial osteotomy of the sagittal split ramus osteotomy.* Journal of Oral and Maxillofacial Surgery, 1991. 49(2): p. 112–116.

[44] Aarabi, M., et al., *Relationship between mandibular anatomy and the occurrence of a bad split upon sagittal split osteotomy.* Journal of Oral and Maxillofacial Surgery, 2014. 72(12): p. 2508–2513.

[45] Falter, B., et al., *Occurrence of bad splits during sagittal split osteotomy.* Oral Surgery, Oral Medicine, Oral Pathology, Oral Radiology, and Endodontology, 2010. 110(4): p. 430–435.

[46] Kriwalsky, M.S., et al., *Risk factors for a bad split during sagittal split osteotomy.* British Journal of Oral and Maxillofacial Surgery, 2008. 46(3): p. 177–179.

[47] Zamiri, B., et al., *Medial cortex fracture patterns after sagittal split osteotomy using short versus long medial cuts: can we obviate bad splits?* International Journal of Oral and Maxillofacial Surgery, 2015.44(7): p. 809–15

[48] Mensink, G., et al., *Bad split during bilateral sagittal split osteotomy of the mandible with separators: a retrospective study of 427 patients.* British Journal of Oral and Maxillofacial Surgery, 2013. 51(6): p. 525–529.

[49] Bouchard, C. and M. Lalancette, *Infections after sagittal split osteotomy: a retrospective analysis of 336 patients.* Journal of Oral and Maxillofacial Surgery, 2015. 73(1): p. 158–161.

[50] Teltzrow, T., et al., *Perioperative complications following sagittal split osteotomy of the mandible.* Journal of Craniomaxillofacial Surgery, 2005. 33(5): p. 307–313.

[51] de Cirugía Ortognática, R.C.D. and U.R. Sistemática, *Condylar resorption after orthognathic surgery: a systematic review.* International Journal of Morphology, 2012. 30(3): p. 1023–1028.

[52] Catherine, Z., P. Breton, and P. Bouletreau, *Condylar resorption after orthognathic surgery: a systematic review.* Revue de stomatologie, de chirurgie maxillo-faciale et de chirurgie orale, 2015.

[53] Valladares-Neto, J., et al., *TMJ response to mandibular advancement surgery: an overview of risk factors.* Journal of Applied Oral Science, 2014. 22(1): p. 2–14.

[54] Panula, K., et al., *Effects of orthognathic surgery on temporomandibular joint dysfunction.* International Journal of Oral & Maxillofacial Surgery, 2000. 29(3): p. 183–187.

[55] Wolford, L.M., O. Reiche-Fischel, and P. Mehra, *Changes in temporomandibular joint dysfunction after orthognathic surgery.* Journal of Oral and Maxillofacial Surgery, 2003. 61(6): p. 655–660; discussion 661.

[56] Al-Riyami, S., S.J. Cunningham, and D.R. Moles, *Orthognathic treatment and temporomandibular disorders: a systematic review. Part 2. Signs and symptoms and meta-analyses.* American Journal of Orthodontics and Dentofacial Orthopedics, 2009. 136(5): p. 626.e1–16, discussion 626–627.

[57] Fernandez-Ferrer, L., et al., *Effects of mandibular setback surgery on upper airway dimensions and their influence on obstructive sleep apnoea — a systematic review.* Journal of Craniomaxillofacial Surgery, 2015. 43(2): p. 248–253.

[58] Hong, J.S., et al., *Three-dimensional changes in pharyngeal airway in skeletal class III patients undergoing orthognathic surgery.* Journal of Craniomaxillofacial Surgery, 2011. 69(11): p. e401–e408.

[59] Gokce, S.M., et al., *Evaluation of pharyngeal airway space changes after bimaxillary orthognathic surgery with a 3-dimensional simulation and modeling program.* American Journal of Orthodontics and Dentofacial Orthopedics, 2014. 146(4): p. 477–492.

[60] Santagata, M., et al., *Effect of orthognathic surgery on the posterior airway space in patients affected by skeletal class III malocclusion.* Journal of Craniomaxillofacial Surgery, 2015. 14(3): p. 682–686.

[61] Al-Moraissi, E.A., et al., *Impact on the pharyngeal airway space of different orthognathic procedures for the prognathic mandible.* International Journal of Oral and Maxillofacial Surgery, 2015. 44(9): p. 1110–1118.

[62] Kawase-Koga, Y., et al., *Complications after intraoral vertical ramus osteotomy: relationship to the shape of the osteotomy line.* International Journal of Oral and Maxillofacial Surgery, 2016. 45(2): p. 200–204.

[63] Ueki, K., et al., *The effects of changing position and angle of the proximal segment after intraoral vertical ramus osteotomy.* International Journal of Oral and Maxillofacial Surgery, 2009. 38(10): p. 1041–1047.

[64] Yamauchi, K., T. Takenobu, and T. Takahashi, *Condylar luxation following bilateral intraoral vertical ramus osteotomy.* Oral Surgery, Oral Medicine, Oral Pathology, Oral Radiology, and Endodontology, 2007. 104(6): p. 747–751.

9

Management of Common Complications in Rhinoplasty and Medical Rhinoplasty

Sebastian Torres and Tito Marianetti

Abstract

Rhinoplasty is considered among the most challenging aesthetic operations because many variables have to be taken into consideration to achieve an optimal aesthetic and functional result. This implies that complications are always waiting around the corner. It is of prime importance to know the main minor and major complications related to the procedure to be able to prevent and treat them promptly when required. Septorhinoplasty is a delicate and difficult procedure, which requires accurate anatomical knowledge and important clinical experience. Nevertheless, complications can affect both inexperienced and expert surgeons. Thus, the most frequent complications of rhinoplasty should be known and adequately prevented when possible.

Keywords: Adverse events, rhinoplasty, complications, rhinofiller, Medical Rhinoplasty

1. Introduction

Some post-operative complications are easily treated, whereas others require multiple reconstructive surgeries and sometimes *restituito ad integrum* (a flawless result) is impossible to obtain. Therefore, the best therapy for complications is prevention. The most frequent complications in rhinoplasty are classified according to their nature as traumatic, respiratory, aesthetic, infective or vascular.

2. Traumatic complications

2.1. L-structure or K-area fracture

During septorhinoplasty, whatever approach is used, two fundamental rules must be kept in mind:

1. Respect the Cottle K area, which is anatomically defined as the intersection of the nasal bones, septum and triangular cartilages.

2. Preserve an adequate dorsal-caudal L structure for support.

Damage to these structures causes an inadequate support of the nasal pyramid and with time causes nasal dorsum collapse and dorsum sill deformity spontaneously or after minor trauma. An adequate dorsal-caudal L structure of at least 1 cm is necessary for structural support to prevent this type of complication. The K area should be addressed with extreme care upon dorsal hump removal. Precise subperiosteal dissection is done above the nasal bones with a Joseph dissector. Incremental dorsal hump reduction with a rasp or osteotomes allows for maneuver control and removes the hard tissue while avoiding damage to the triangular cartilages or nasal bones.

Treatment of L-structure fractures of the septum includes the use of robust reconstructive spreader grafts on the dorsal segment and columellar strut grafts on the caudal segment. Septal cartilage grafts are preferred when available; otherwise, conchae or costal cartilage grafts are necessary.

Repair of K-area damage and triangular cartilage detachment from the nasal bones is more complex. If a small residue of cephalic cartilage remains, reattachment of the triangular cartilages is possible with non-resorbable sutures. Otherwise, holes are drilled in the nasal bone to anchor stitches of the triangular cartilages. Permanent surgical sutures (Nylon 4.0) are preferred over Kirchner metal wire, as proposed by other authors, given the fact that the skin is extremely thin in this area and a greater incidence of infection, irregularities and transcutaneous translucency can be expected with the latter technique.

2.2. Dental trauma

Hypoanesthesia of the superior central incisors and palatal premaxilla is frequently noted in the post-operative period after septorhinoplasty. This is due to the fact that the incisive nerve, before exiting in the oral cavity through the homonymous canal, lies on the maxillary crest at the base of the nasal septum. This complication frequently arises when septal dislocations close to the anterior nasal spine, nasal septum cartilage resections or anterior nasal spine remodeling procedures are done. Spontaneous resolution of the hypoesthesia is expected for the majority, and sensitivity is reestablished in a variable period between 1 week and 6 months. In the case of abnormal vascular support of superior anterior incisors or long teeth roots, a direct damage to the superior central incisors is possible; this can cause pulpitis or abnormal pigmentation. Prompt dental evaluation and endodontic therapy are advised, if necessary, before intrinsic pigmentation occurs or more complex and expensive prosthetic therapies are needed.

2.3. Intracranial complications

Intracranial complications include rhino-liquoral fistulas and anosmia. **Rhino-liquoral fistulas** are among the major post-rhinoplasty complications.

Given the fact that the superior portion of the septal cartilage is directly abutting the cribriform lamina of the ethmoid and is the direct continuation of this structure, an understanding of why this severe complication is not that uncommon is apparent.

Septoplasty is a delicate phase of the procedure. Very often, surgeons treat the septum aggressively by grabbing the bony portion with Weil forceps and attempting to break or remove the tissue through rotatory movements. Prevention of rhino-liquoral fistulas consists of an accurate and delicate septum dissection, particularly with regard to the superior bone portion. Before pulling a fragment, adequate dissection and freeing is necessary. The clinical symptomatology of rhino-liquoral fistulas includes rhinorrhea and positional cephalus. Diagnosis is confirmed through beta-2 transferrin presence in the fluid, specifically the cerebrospinal fluid.

Such complication requires hospitalization, lumbar drainage positioning by a neurosurgeon and eventual multilayer nasal endoscopic fistula repair.

Anosmia is fortunately very seldom observed due to the damage of the olfactory bulb. Most frequently, this condition is secondary to a persistent respiratory nasal obstructive pathology.

2.4. Orbital complications

Orbital complications related to septorhinoplasty are extremely rare and include blindness and epiphora. Blindness has been reported in some cases and is related to turbinate or nasal dorsum steroid injections. The etiopathogenesis described involves an embolic occlusion of the central retinal artery. Other cases due to vasoconstrictor injections in the septum and turbinates, being the etiology of a spastic response on the central retinal artery, have been described [1–3].

These unfortunate complications are hard to predict and impossible to resolve. For this reason, prevention is done by avoiding steroid infiltration in the turbinates and aspiration prior to injection and injecting a small quantity when treating the dorsum. Epiphora is an extremely rare complication after rhinoplasty. Lateral osteotomies are generally safe if executed in a standard manner. Damage to the lacrimal ducts is possible when the osteotomy direction is incorrect or when motorized instruments or saws are used. It is frequently clinically confused with paralateronasal edema. Spontaneous resolution is often verified, although sporadic cases require dacryocystorhinostomy for complete resolution [4, 5].

3. Respiratory complications

3.1. Internal nasal valve dysfunction

Internal nasal valve dysfunction is a frequent complication secondary to old school destructive rhinoplasty. The principal cause is over-resection of the lateral cartilages during hump removal. The internal nasal valve angle is formed by the confluence of the nasal septum medially and lateral cartilages externally; its normal value is around 15° [6].

A reduction in this value determines impairment in airway flow. More severe than an excessive resection of the triangular cartilages is scarring in the internal valve area due to transmucosal disjunction of the septum from the triangular cartilages; fortunately, this is an old and discarded technique. Patients with a non-deviated septum are referred for treatment of severe nasal respiratory problems. Moreover, in addition to this severe functional defect, a dorsal inverted V deformity appears after the resolution of the surgical edema due to inferomedial collapse of the triangular cartilages [7].

The remedy for this type of complication is the placement of a spreader graft, whatever the type (auto, mini or classic) and source (septum, concha or rib). The important technical detail is to place the graft so as to raise and reposition the collapsed triangular cartilages and return internal nasal valve function, augmenting the cross-sectional area.

Classic spreader grafts are longitudinal grafts placed in a subperichondrial pocket and fixed to the triangular cartilages and the septum through non-resorbable sutures.

Spreader grafts also allow straightening of a cephalic deviated septum, reconstruction of an open roof deformity or improvement of dorsal aesthetic lines [8].

Auto-spreader grafts are obtained from the triangular cartilages after mucosal dissection and then partially cut and folded medially over themselves; this maneuver is very difficult to perform in secondary cases due to prior over-resection of the cartilages. On the other hand, mini-spreader grafts are obtained from the cephalic portion of the alar cartilages but due to their reduced dimensions are seldom useful for severe reconstruction [9].

3.2. Nasal septal perforation

The etiology of septal perforation is diverse and may be iatrogenic, which is most often the case, due to cocaine abuse, infections, trauma and granulomatous diseases. With subperichondrial septum dissection, caution should be taken not to trespass the mucoperichondrial flaps. It is advisable to start with the easier side to grant integrity in at least one side. When both mucosal flaps are damaged bilaterally, an iatrogenic septal perforation will be produced.

The symptomatology of septal perforation includes crusts, recurrent bleeding, whistling or inspiratory rumors and nasal respiratory obstruction. The more anterior the perforation is, the greater the associated disturbance.

The most ancient solution for the problem was the use of silicone septal buttons, which are less popular among patients nowadays.

Diverse septal perforation repair techniques have been described, with the most effective ones being from Kridel and Castelnuovo [10, 11]. Kridel described an open approach for the provision of sliding superior (from the internal nasal valve region) and inferior (from the nasal floor and inferior turbinate) mucoperichondrial flaps. Castelnuovo reported an endoscopic approach for an intranasal septal mucosal pedunculated flap to the ethmoidal arteries, which is rotated to obtain defect closure. Both techniques grant a high success rate.

Whatever the case, it is proper to prevent septal perforation and if verified to take time to repair the mucoperichondrial flaps properly. Allotting an additional 10 minutes at the primary surgery is better than performing 3 hours of revision surgery for perforation closure.

3.3. External nasal valve dysfunction

The external nasal valve is an area defined three-dimensionally by the inferior turbinate head, caudal portion of the triangular cartilages, cephalic portion of the alar cartilages and septum. The most common source of post-rhinoplasty dysfunction is related to an excessive resection of lateral crura of the alar cartilages.

This condition is occasionally seen when an attempt to reduce nose tip dimensions is sought at all costs, not leaving enough alar cartilage to support the nasal ala.

Nasal alar collapse can be dynamic if it manifests only during inspiration (forced or not) or static in more severe cases if it is verified at rest. The minimum alar cartilage dimension to preserve varies according to the intrinsic consistency of the cartilage and it is not the same for all patients. Nevertheless, a minimum of 4–5 mm should be kept and old risky, interruptive approaches should be avoided.

Multiple techniques have been described to treat this complication, namely, alar spreader grafts, lateral crura repositioning, alar spanning grafts, barrel roll technique, lateral crura strut grafts and alar batten grafts. Alar batten grafts are the most frequently used, but every case should be analyzed individually and treated accordingly with the most indicated technique [12].

External nasal valve compromise is also verified after maneuvers that cause narinal stenosis. This condition is seen, for example, when a sloppy adaptation of the vestibular skin occurs after rhinoplasty due to a lack of closing sutures in the area, infection or abnormal scarring. Another cause is represented by excessive alar base wedge resection.

Corrections in these cases are complex and foresee the use of local flaps and Z-plasties, but in the majority of cases, auricular composite grafts are necessary to replenish the lack of previously excised tissue.

Residual anterior septal deviations and turbinate hypertrophy can cause external nasal valve dysfunction. Residual anterior septal deviations require surgical revision with a more precise septoplasty. Inferior turbinate hypertrophy is very frequent, especially in allergic patients. In these cases, medical therapy is advised with local steroids and systemic antihistamines, discouraging continuous surgical retouching [13].

Turbinoseptal synechiae (adherences) can also produce external nasal valve stenosis, although they can appear even more posteriorly in the nasal fossae. Silicone splints should be used and kept in place long enough to allow re-epithelization of the turbinate and septum to prevent turbinoseptal synechiae when mucosal lacerations occur.

3.4. Sinusitis

Sinusitis is rare as a post-rhinoplasty complication, but it can become apparent if unrecognized predisposing conditions are present.

The medial meatus protected by the middle turbinate represents the common drainage path for the ducts of paranasal sinuses. Ethmoidal anterior, frontal and maxillary sinuses all drain at this level.

Medial turbinate lateralization maneuvers are extremely dangerous as they may cause rhino-liquoral fistulas and compromise normal paranasal sinus function.

If predisposing conditions are present, the presence of concha bullosa may predispose a patient to post-rhinoplasty sinusitis. It is advisable to assess pre-operative nasal and paranasal sinus CT scans that will give valuable information regarding septal deviation and turbinate hypertrophy and identify sinusal alterations suitable to be treated during the surgery through functional endoscopic sinus surgery (FESS) to avoid this complication.

4. Aesthetic complications

4.1. Supratip deformity (polly beak)

Post-operative deformity of the supratip nasal area that assumes a convex shape in relation to the nasal dorsum can have two sources: cartilaginous tissue or scar tissue. Cartilaginous polly beaks are caused by an insufficient resection of the inferior third of the dorsal septum in proximity to the septal angle. Scar tissue polly beaks, on the other hand, are more frequent in cases with sebaceous skin and are due to hypertrophic scarring of the subcutaneous tissue of the supratip region.

Prevention of cartilaginous supratips relies on meticulous assessment of an adequate relation between the dorsum and nasal tip. Normally, the distance between the level of tip-defining points and septal angle is about 6–8 mm, but it is based on the surgeon's experience to define the magnitude [14].

Supratip scarring is more difficult to prevent. Supratip empty spaces that may fill with blood and further scar tissue should be avoided.

Compressive bandaging of the supratip area for 4–5 weeks is of prime importance to reduce the dead space and prevent polly beak deformity from scarring.

The remedy for supratip scarring is based on local steroid injections; they are very effective if done properly with regard to timing and modality. Triamcinolone acetonide (Kenacort, 40 mg/ml injectable suspension) is the steroid of choice. Dosage should be triamcinolone 1–2 mg applied early (2–3 weeks after the surgery) if a tendency for supratip deformity is perceived and not repeated before a 2-month interval. The effect of the therapy is seen in the following 2 months post injection. The injections should be in a deep plane and never intradermal.

Superficial injection causes cutaneous atrophy, telangiectasia, depressions, color modifications and underlying cartilage visibility [15].

Cartilaginous supratips and non-responders with scar-based supratips are treated with revision surgery. An in-depth analysis of tip-dorsum relation and the use of tip-defining grafts (onlays and shields) are useful to avoid recidivism.

4.2. Dorsal irregularities

The nasal dorsum is the region more prone to unexpected and unwanted surprises after a rhinoplasty. It is very difficult for the surgeon to ensure that no dorsum unevenness remains at the end of surgery and that the end result is smooth and with no imperfections in the majority. Nevertheless, months or years after the surgery, it is difficult to find an operated nose that does not show some dorsal irregularities at least upon palpation. The reason for this is that surgical edema will hide small irregularities and mask an adequate palpation evaluation of dorsum smoothness. With time, as nasal tissue swelling disappears, irregularities start to show [16].

Dorsal deformities are among the most common causes of revision rhinoplasty. They are mostly due to excessive or inadequate hump removal, remnant fragments after removal, asymmetric resections, inadequate graft modeling or fixation and dislocation.

Open rhinoplasty can reduce the frequency of these imperfections as it allows for direct vision of the dorsum. Another tip to reduce the percentage of these complications is to perform dorsal index palpation with the surgical gloves wetted with normal saline, augmenting sensitivity for the surgeon. Profuse cleansing and washing of the dorsal area under the skin envelope before suturing is imperative as it eliminates small cartilage residues and bony fragments, avoiding future irregularities.

Avoiding dorsal irregularities in patients with thin skin is still very difficult. In these cases, it may be advisable to use dorsal augmenting materials. These can be autologous (temporal fascia, perichondrium graft), heterologous (equine or bovine pericardium membranes) or alloplastic (Gore-Tex). Autologous materials are preferable due to the lower incidence of infections associated with them; however, at the dorsum level, the risk of infection or extrusion is very small even for non-autologous materials [17].

4.3. Tip deviations and irregularities

Tip deviations and irregularities are among the most common causes of revision rhinoplasty and are more prevalent in the closed approach. They include depressions, irregularities, asymmetries and lateral crura collapse. They can appear due to faulty techniques, excessive or asymmetric lateral crura resections, incorrect graft positioning or scarring [18, 19].

Another particularly anti-aesthetic condition is an altered tip projection, either hyperprojection or hypoprojection. Nose tip deformities often manifest a long time after the surgery (1 or 2 years after). In fact, the nose tip is the last region to swell down in the post-operative period.

Prevention of this complication relies on knowledge of tip supportive mechanics and the tripod theory as well as attention to avoid disruptive or destructive techniques. Nevertheless, the most important factors are still expertise and respecting aesthetic proportions that will grant good results in the long term. Revision rhinoplasty is surely easier and predictable if done via an open approach, but this also depends on the skills and experience of the surgeon [20].

4.4. Skin necrosis

Nasal skin necrosis is among the worst complications that can occur during a septorhinoplasty. It is mainly caused by vascular damage in the vessels that supply the nose tip. Rarely, it can present due to excessive dressing compression. Most frequently, it appears after damage in the lateral nasal arteries due to an incorrect plane of dissection or following excessive nose tip fat tissue reduction, in an attempt to reduce its size.

A new source of skin necrosis of increasing prevalence is the post-operative use of dermal fillers at the nasal pyramid, nasolabial folds or paranasal region to camouflage irregularities. This outcome is more frequently verified when the filler is delivered with needles that may cause direct vessel damage and intravascular occlusion or indirect vascular compression, jeopardizing tip vascularity.

Some rules should be respected to prevent this complication:

1. Avoid injecting fillers with sharp needles (preferably blunt tip cannulas) in paranasal areas.

2. Dissect the nasal tissues attached to the cartilaginous framework without getting superficial.

3. Avoid defatting techniques of the nose tip or reduce it to a minimum.

4. Avoid firm and tight dressings, especially in revision cases.

5. Limit alar wedge resections under the alar crease.

Treatment of skin necrosis is very complex and ranges from conservative approaches (such as second-intention wound healing) to complex reconstruction procedures with local, regional or free flaps. Whatever the approach, skin tropism and elasticity are a primary goal before intending more complex repair. The latter procedure can be achieved through platelet-rich plasma and micro-lipofilling sessions.

5. Infective complications

Rhinoplasty infections are not frequent, probably due to the natural protective mechanisms of the nasal mucosa. Nevertheless, the myriad of infective cases can be very vast and go from small subcutaneous cellulitis due to infected sutures to severe cavernous sinus thrombosis.

Local skin or mucosal infections are treated with local and systemic antibiotics. Abscesses may affect the dorsum, tip or septum, with septal abscess being the most dangerous, and they should be promptly drained; septal abscess can appear from an undiagnosed septal hematoma that can evolve to a septal perforation if not treated promptly.

High fever, meningeal signs, nausea, vomiting and hypotension are suggestive signs of a severe infection, such as cavernous sinus thrombosis. If the diagnosis is suspected, nasal tampons should be removed immediately (especially if placed several days before) and secretions should be sent for cultural and bacteriological analysis, with the most frequent germ involved being *Staphylococcus aureus*. Patients should be hospitalized and systemic antibiotics should be initiated promptly.

Prophylactic antibiotics in rhinoplasty are a controversial topic but nonetheless highly indicated by the majority of surgeons.

6. Vascular complications

Vascular complications include septal hematoma and epistaxis.

6.1. Septal hematoma

Septal hematoma can occur secondary to trauma or surgery and is a serious complication. Its symptomatology includes nasal obstruction, pain and, occasionally, fever. Anterior rhinoscopy reveals a septal mass that occludes one or both nasal fossae. Immediate therapy is indicated and consists of hematoma drainage, nasal tampons to impede recidivism and proper antibiotic therapy to avoid abscess transformation.

Septal abscesses can evolve to mucosal and/or cartilage necrosis and septal perforation varying in dimension and location according to the underlying infection [21].

6.2. Epistaxis

Bleeding in rhinoplasty patients post-operatively is normal if limited, whereas it can become a complication if profuse or continuous. The condition is more frequent in at-risk patients on anticoagulants or platelet anti-aggregating agents. In these cases, prior consultation with a hematologist and a cardiologist is advisable, and oral clot-altering drugs should be discontinued and subcutaneous LMW heparin initiated several days before the surgery. All patients should be advised to discontinue NSAID or aspirin intake at least 2 weeks prior to operation.

A precise and delicate technique during surgery is desirable to avoid vascular problems. During septoplasty, for example, it is important to avoid mucosal flap lacerations to minimize bleeding. A nasal septum mattress suture can be useful to prevent bleeding and septal hematoma. Turbinate cautery should be gentle. An open technique allows for direct vision and hemostasis of bleeding vessels during the procedure. Epistaxis therapy includes 60° head elevation, nasal packing and gentle nares pressure for 10–15 minutes. Severe epistaxis can require an emergency endoscopic procedure to coagulate the sphenopalatine septal and lateral branches.

7. Medical rhinoplasty

Medical rhinoplasty was first described by Braccini and Dohan Ehrenfest [22] in 2008. The concept, although highly polemical and refused by rhinoplasty surgeons at its onset, developed popularity among aesthetic patients due to its minimally invasive characteristics, with minimal or no downtime and pleasing aesthetic improvements.

The term *medical rhinoplasty* (particularly, *rhinofiller*) is defined as the application of dermal fillers in the external or internal nasal area to modify or improve aesthetics or functionality. It is especially suitable for patients with minor aesthetic or functional concerns that are refractory to surgery [23–26]. It may be combined with the use of botulinum toxin injections around the nose to enhance the results. The procedure is currently a frequent request in aesthetic practice, and many physicians perform it systematically. Nevertheless, it should be considered that it is an advanced technique and should only be attempted by expert practitioners due to the potential for devastating vascular complications [27]. Local anatomical knowledge and advanced technical skills are required to achieve successful and safe corrections.

7.1. Rhinofiller

Rhinofiller specifically involves the infiltration of a dermal filler to modify external or internal nasal structures for aesthetic or functional purposes. Since its introduction in 2008, many temporary and permanent substances have been used to achieve the desired corrections. Successful application mandates adequate anatomical knowledge of the related structures.

Proper patient selection is important to achieve good results. Exclusion criteria include severe nasal airway impairment, permanent filler in the area, history of ischemic/thrombotic events or known hypercoagulability, local infection and recent trauma.

Before the procedure, nasal analysis should be performed clinically and photographically to define needed corrections.

Areas of potential correction include dorsal aesthetic lines, the dorsum, minor hump camouflage, radix enhancement, tip rotation and projection and base augmentation. Details are shown in **Figure 11**.

Functionally, in selected cases, the use of fillers can be useful to augment the aperture of the internal nasal valve as a volumetric spreader graft.

Morphing simulations are advisable before treatment in order to give patients an indication of the post-treatment outcomes, explain the procedure and establish common goals. In addition, specific, informed consent should be properly discussed and obtained.

7.1.1. Technique

Treatments are typically performed with medium-viscosity hyaluronic acid (HA) fillers under local anesthetic (lidocaine intradermal vesicles applied using a 0.3 ml syringe with a 32G needle) with the aid of a 25G (0.5 mm) × 4 cm blunt-tip disposable cannula, manually bent, maintaining sterility at all times, in order to obtain better compliance of the shapes and silhouette within the nasal area. The distribution of material should be performed as required to follow the treatment plan. Tip refinements can be sporadically carried out through needle infiltration with extreme care.

The specific pattern of anesthetic peripheral blocks and filler infiltration is shown in **Figure 12**.

Generally, the patient satisfaction rate with this correction is very high and, due to the scarce muscular activity in the nose, corrections with Hyaluronic acid dermal fillers last more than 1 year and in many cases even 2 years. A clinical case of rhinofiller is described in **Figures 13** and **14**.

8. Discussion

The nasal area is composed of different interacting tissues, such as the skin, subcutaneous tissue, muscle, bone, cartilage and mucosa, which come together to form a normal, functional and aesthetically pleasing nose. To make things more complicated, there is also a vascular anatomy formed by two main circuits, namely, the supratrochlear and dorsal arteries and the facial circuit that includes the superior labial and angular arteries, all of which are anastomosed in the tip. This has been the subject of recent interest and study because it is believed that a proper technique and anatomical knowledge are of prime importance in order to avoid vascular complications [28–30]. Facial vascular complications were first described in 1991 after collagen injections in the glabellar area [31]. The reported incidence of Nicolau syndrome or embolia cutis medicamentosa (ECM) following glabellar treatments is 9/10,000 procedures (0.09%). The known risk factors associated with this catastrophic event are a high syringe piston pressure, a highly vascularized territory and previously traumatized tissue. The first of these factors can be mitigated using fluid materials of low viscosity. Unfortunately, the entire facial region, especially the nasal area, is considered highly vascularized and many reports of paranasal vascular complications, which vary from mild symptoms of pain and skin color changes to necrosis and even bilateral blindness, have been published [32–41]. The pathophysiology of ECM is an intravascular injection that advances in a retrograde mode to a distant area and, through changes in blood pressure, arrives at a distant vessel and causes a vascular complication. The resulting symptoms vary according to the physiology of the vessel that is compromised; affliction of arteries leads to pallor, whereas occlusion of veins manifests as livedo reticularis. According to the author's experience, there is a second mechanism of vascular compromise in the nose known as *compartmental syndrome*. Due to the low elasticity of the nasal skin (especially after surgical rhinoplasty), there is a chance of producing indirect vascular compromise due to mechanical obstruction when large amounts of filler are positioned, even in the absence of intravascular injection. The former, together with the altered anatomy and possible iatrogenic vascular damage, makes these corrections particularly tricky in this patient setting. Vascular complications can range from mild to severe and therefore prompt recognition and treatment are crucial. Oral aspirin, nitrate cream 2%, heat, massages and intralesional hyaluronidase have all been proven to be beneficial. The author has also used intralesional heparin mesotherapy with good results (unpublished observations). In severe, unresponsive cases, prostaglandin E_1 (alprostadil) treatment can sometimes limit the extent of the damage. For the remaining scar tissue, occasionally complex reconstruction procedures are necessary [42, 43], although the recent use of stem cells has shown promising results [44]. All of the above have determined nasal augmentation with dermal fillers to be particularly challenging, and mastery of the correct technique is of utmost importance in order to achieve good results and reduce the incidence of adverse reactions. Important factors to consider include the following:

- **Patient selection:** Proper patient selection is vital in order to achieve a good outcome. Rule out individuals with unrealistic expectations and treat post-rhinoplasty patients with extreme care.

- **Materials:** A good technique begins with selection of the correct materials. Only temporary or autologous materials (fat) should be used in the nose. Among temporary materials, HA is the best option because it causes no fibrotic changes in the subcutaneous tissue, such as those that can occur with calcium hydroxyapatite. Moderate-viscosity HA is preferred due to the lower piston pressure in the syringe associated with it.

- **Correct amount of material:** Never exceed the correct quantity of filler used in the nose. It is always better to undercorrect and then repeat as needed. A good safety measure is to stay within 1 ml of filler per session. Remember that the pressure of the material can induce vascular problems even without being intravascular. Place the fingers to position and maintain the product in the target area to avoid migration. Small amounts of material should be placed using low infiltrative pressure and few passes in a retrograde infiltration fashion.

- **Cryotherapy:** It is always wise to favor vasoconstriction in order to limit bruising and edema and reduce intravascular compromise.

- **Cannula, manually curved:** The use of atraumatic cannulas permits gentle dissection of the tissues, reduces the trauma and risks of intravascular injection and delivers the material through a laminar flux that guarantees evenness. The manually curved feature allows for perfect shape compatibility with the nasal dorsum. The use of local anesthetic vesicles and needle skin penetration prior to cannula entry limits pain, trauma and vascular compromise.

- **Needles:** Extreme caution should be used when injecting with needles around the nose; their use should be limited to retouches or refinements and only by very experienced physicians. Perform tunnels (visible entry and exit points created with the needle being used) and allow material to exit if needed. The most risky areas are the tip, glabella, canine fossa and columellar base. Avoid bolus techniques in these regions and inject only when *coming out*. It is preferable to use medium-sized needles and inject into the deep or intermediate plane. Prior aspiration is not useful.

- **Improve; do not attempt a perfect outcome:** This technique should be considered part of the armamentarium of every aesthetic surgeon but not used as a single instrument. Whenever we want to completely correct a surgical deformity with fillers, we get into possible complications.

- **Planning and discussion of potential complications:** It is essential to obtain proper informed consent. Frequently, patients are ill-informed about this procedure and have often read that it is extremely easy and free of risks. Establish a good relationship based on truth and trust with your patient. Morphing software can be of great help in this phase to help communicate with patients and establish common goals; underpromise and overdeliver.

- **Analyze the columellar labial angle:** Analysis of this feature allows for objectivity of the outcome and even the most critical patients will be able to appreciate the improvement.

- **Available kit for potential ECM:** If you intend to treat the nose with dermal fillers, you should be prepared to handle the complications as well.

9. Conclusions

The use of dermal fillers around the nose, although an advanced technique with potentially severe adverse events, is a powerful tool that can be used with a great deal of satisfaction and safety for the benefit of patients who wish to achieve aesthetic or functional improvements without a surgical procedure. The risks and benefits should always be considered and discussed, and complications should be prevented and promptly treated if necessary.

9.1. Nasal botulinum toxin

The onset of the neurotoxin in aesthetics revolutionized the treatment of dynamic facial dynamic wrinkles, producing a reversible paralysis that allows overlying tissues to relax and aesthetically to be flattened and raised. The use of botulinum toxin around the nose differs from the typically recommended indications of the superior facial third, being considered an advanced and off-label technique.

The use of botulinum toxin in the nose is useful in hypermotile noses that typically move with mimic expression. The complications related to this technique are not as severe as those associated with the use of rhinofiller as they are reversible and do not affect nose vascularity. Complications include pain, bruising, swelling, asymmetries, short-lasting effect and resistance. The duration of the corrections is limited (3–4 months) and action takes 2–10 days to establish, but it may enhance the results obtained with a rhinofiller as it removes muscular action and tension over the nasal region. Deep punctures at a muscular level are necessary.

The following muscles suitable for treatment around the nose are as follows:

- The **nasalis transverse muscle** is responsible for the wrinkling in the radix paranasal region known as *bunny lines*. Treatment typically requires 1–2 U per side 1 mm above the angular vessels at the lateral aspect of the radix.

- The **levator anguli oris alaeque nasi muscle** is responsible for gummy smiles. Treatment requires 2–5 U per side at the intersection of the nasolabial fold and the alar region.

- The **depressor septi nasi muscle** is responsible for hypermotile nose tips and an acute columellar labial angle. Treatment requires 1–2 U at the base of the columella.

- The **alar nasalis muscle** acts together with the depressor septi nasi muscle to lower the tip projection and restrict the nasal aperture. Treatment requires 1–2 U per side at the midpoint of the alar area.

A summary of these muscles and their corresponding treatment doses is given in **Figures 15**.

10. Clinical case patients

10.1. Clinical case patient 1

A 28-year-old female patient who previously underwent destructive septorhinoplasty with excessive resection of the alar and triangular cartilages presented to us with an inverted V deformity, right nasal alar collapse, tip asymmetry and a deformed dorsum sill.

Revision rhinoplasty was done using an open approach and harvesting right concha cartilage grafts. Tip de-projection, right lateral reconstruction and bilateral spreader graft positioning were performed (**Figures 1–4**).

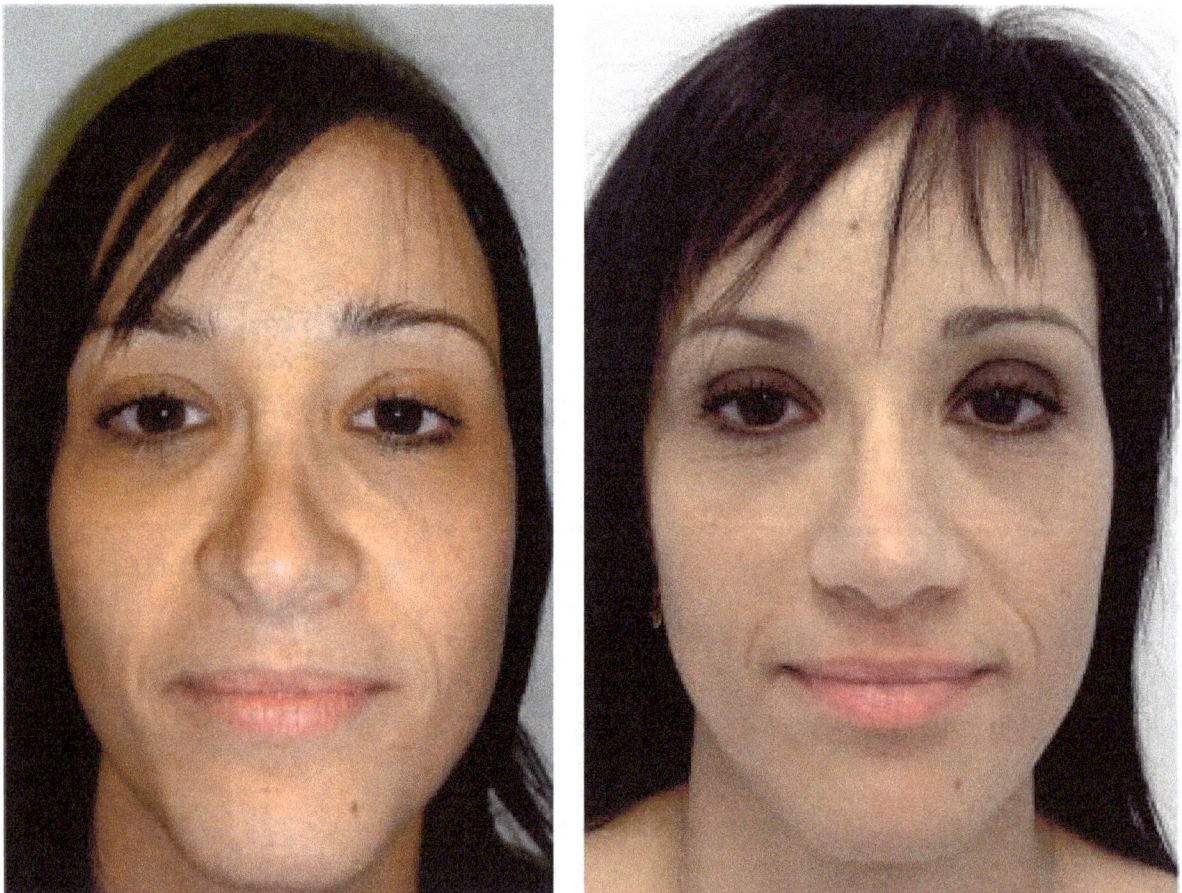

Figure 1. Clinical case 1: Before (right) and after (left) images.

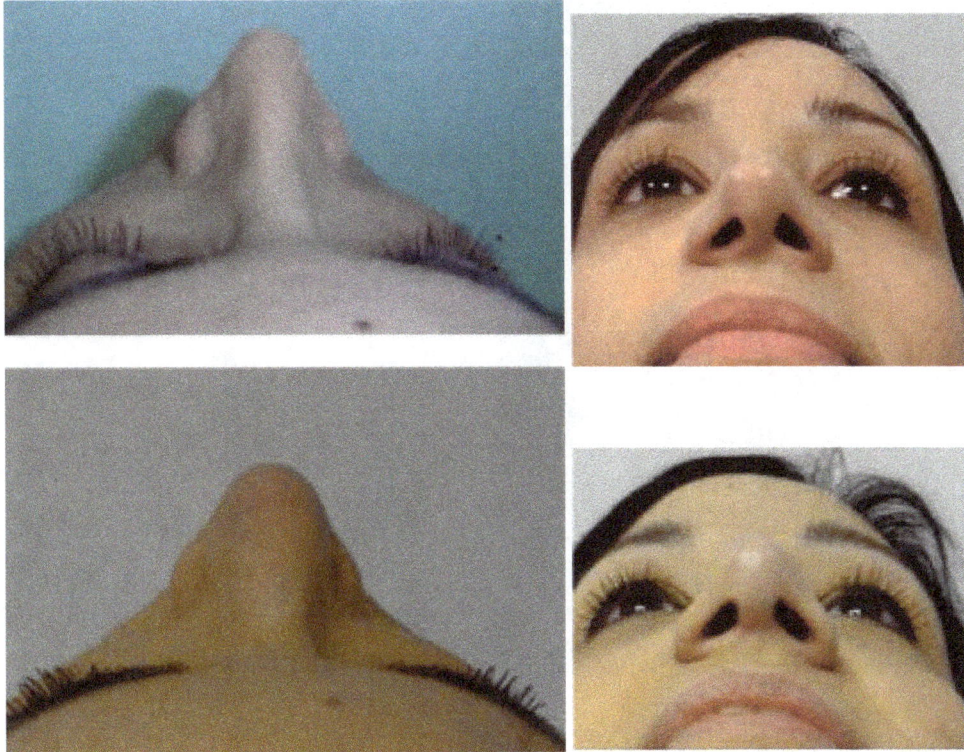

Figure 2. Clinical case 1: Before (upper) and after (below) images.

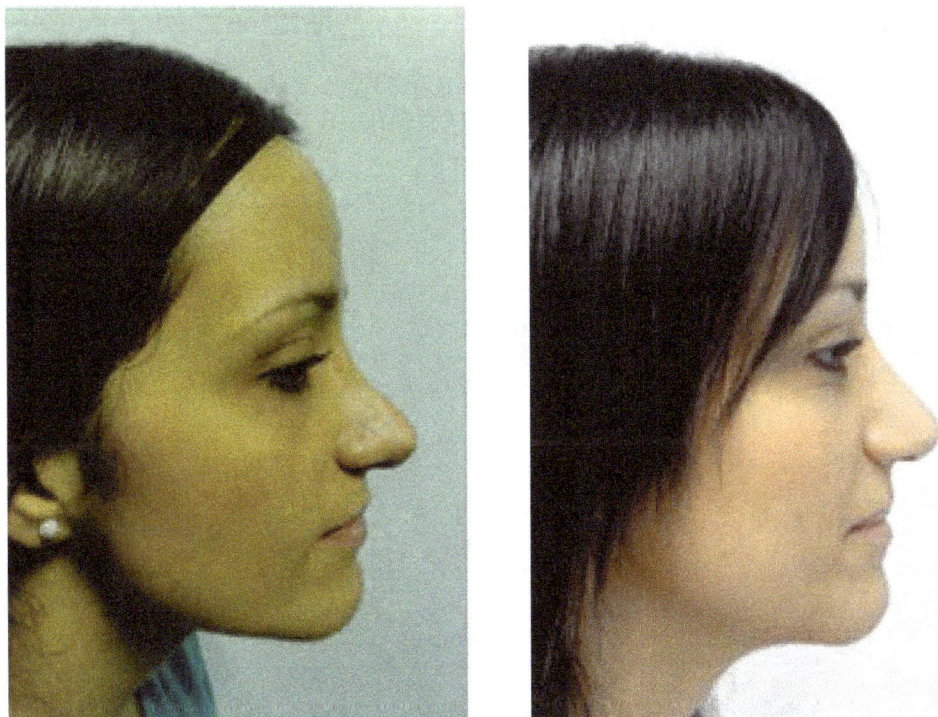

Figure 3. Clinical case 1: Before (left) and after (right) images, lateral view.

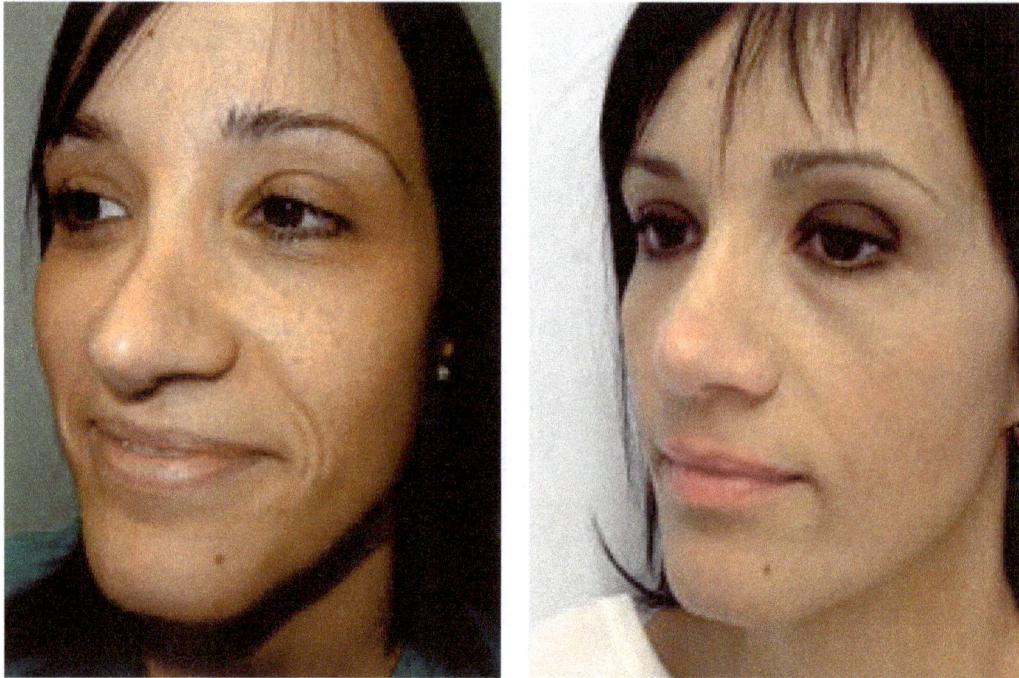

Figure 4. Clinical case 1: Before (left) and after (right) images, oblique view.

10.2. Clinical case patient 2

A 42-year-old female patient who previously underwent septorhinoplasty presented to us with dorsal irregularity, tip asymmetry and a 3 cm diameter anterior septal perforation.

Reconstructive procedure was performed using an open approach and the Kridel septal perforation closure technique. Regularization of the dorsum and tip symmetrization was done (**Figures 5–8**).

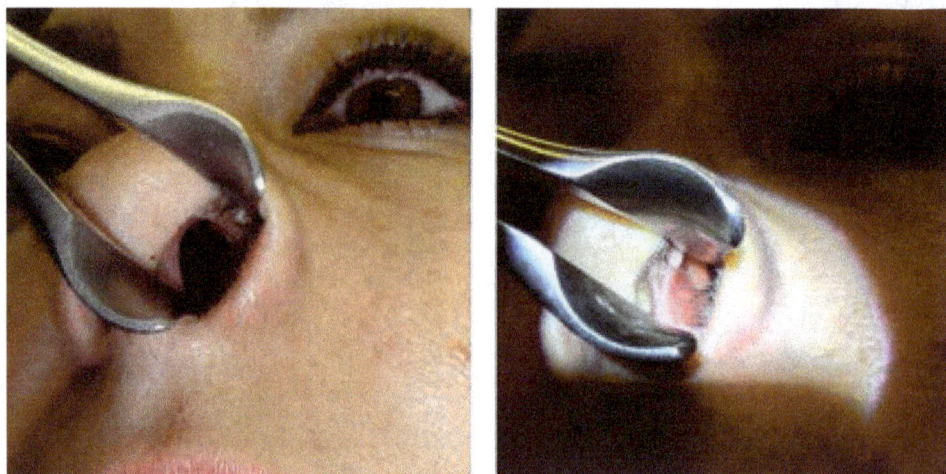

Figure 5. Clinical case 2: Septal perforation.

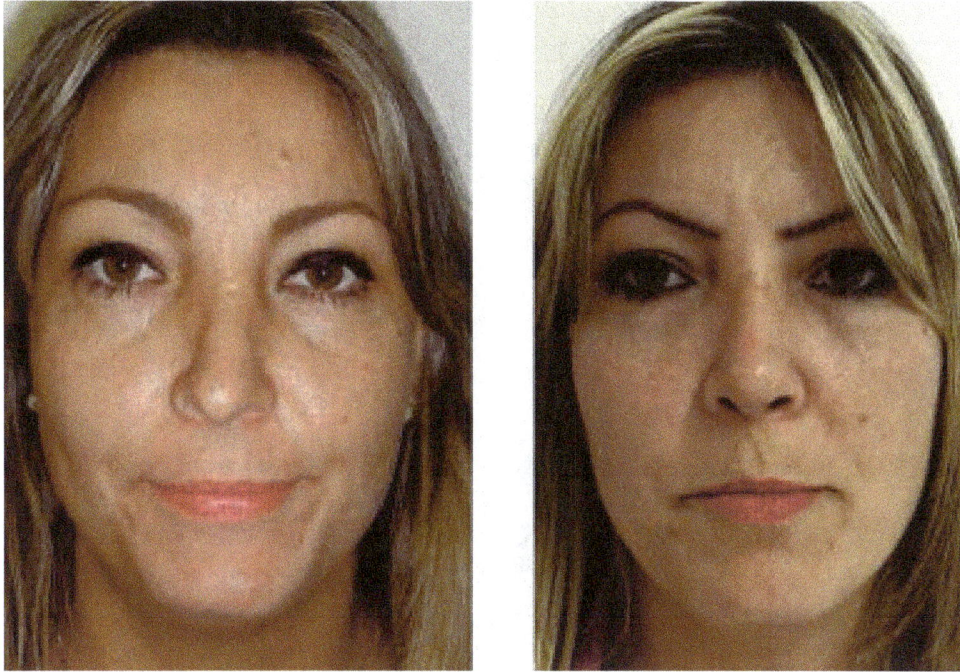

Figure 6. Clinical case 2: Before (right) and after (left) images.

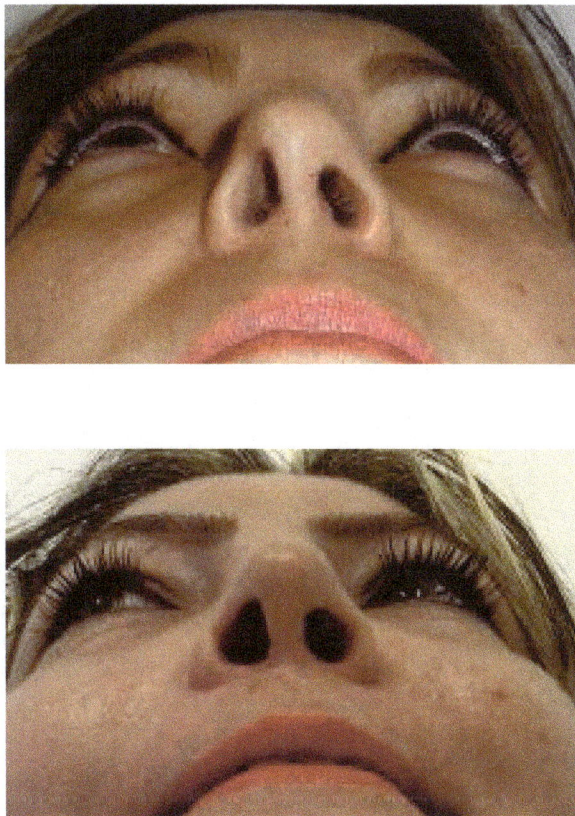

Figure 7. Clinical case 2: Before (upper) and after (lower) images, basal view.

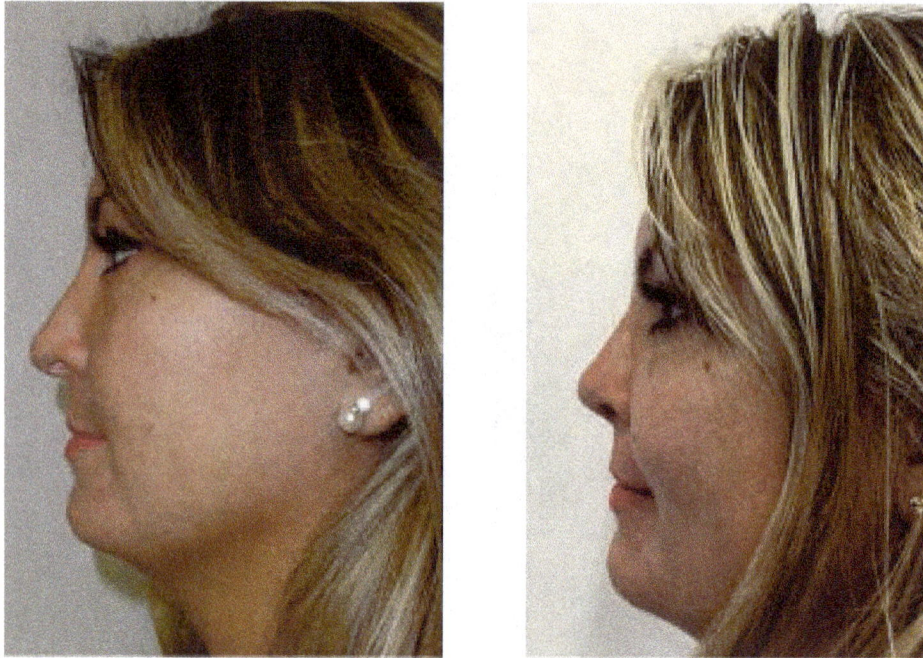

Figure 8. Clinical case 2: Before (right) and after (left) images, lateral view.

10.3. Clinical case patient 3

We also report the case of nasal lipofilling for iatrogenic skin necrosis post-rhinoplasty and filler use in a 22-year-old female patient who previously underwent open rhinoplasty and received several steroids and filler (HA) treatments in the post-operative period until the nose tip, alar cartilages, caudal septum and anterior nasal spine vascularity were jeopardized. The patient was referred with severe scarring and low skin elasticity. She refused reconstruction with a forehead flap. Our treatment plan was initiated with PRP mesotherapy to the nasal region through a dermic pen device. Successive nasal micro-lipofilling sessions (×4) enhanced with a 20% mix of PRP significantly improved skin quality and elasticity for further reconstructive steps (**Figure 9**).

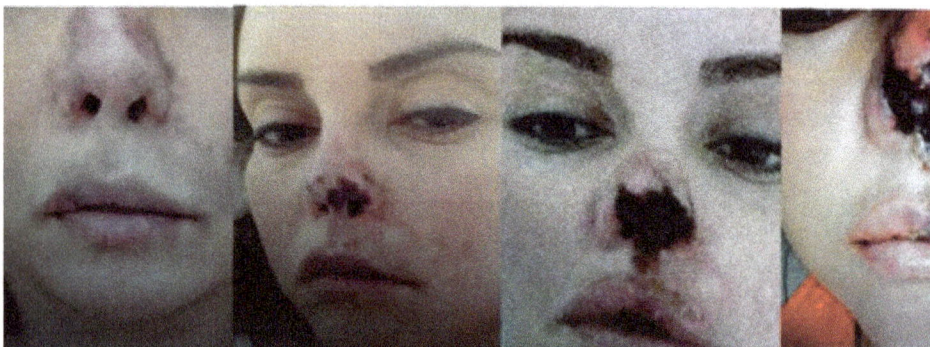

Figure 9. Clinical case 3: Dramatic ischemic progression due to fillers and steroid injections post-rhinoplasty courtesy of Dr Sebastian Torres.

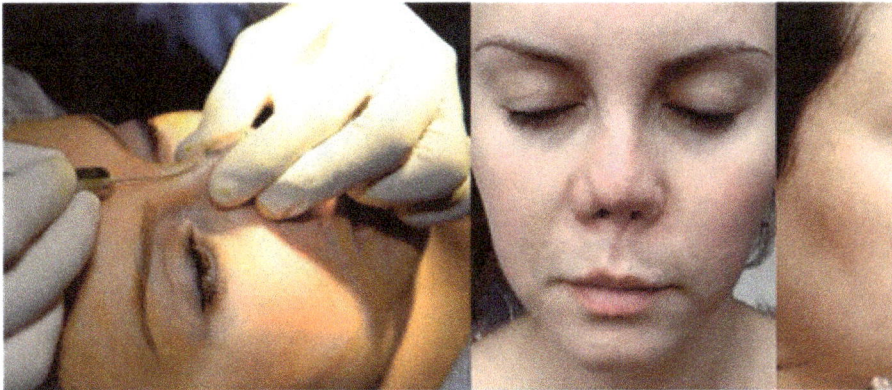

Figure 10. Clinical case 3: Micro-lipofilling technique (left) and post-operative (12 months) reconstructive procedures (center and right) courtesy of Dr Sebastian Torres.

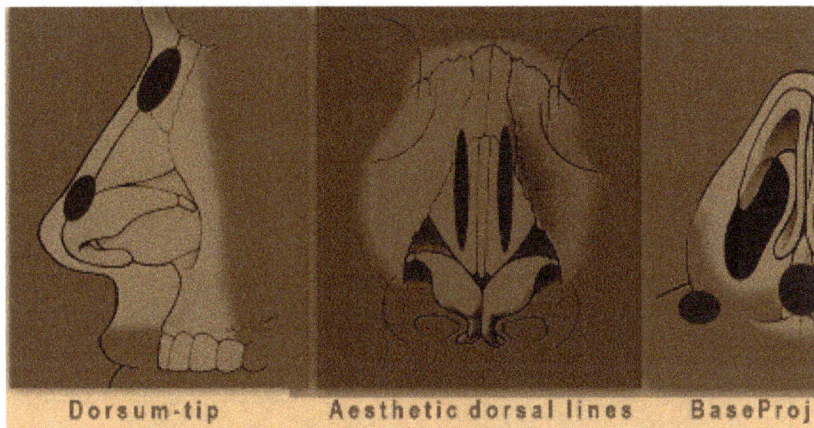

Figure 11. Rhinofiller main treatment areas.

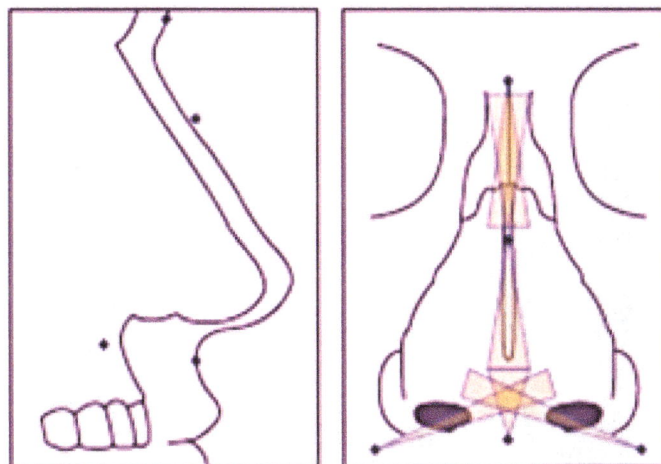

Figure 12. Rhinofiller injection technique. Spots indicate the entry point for cannula; orange triangles indicate material distribution.

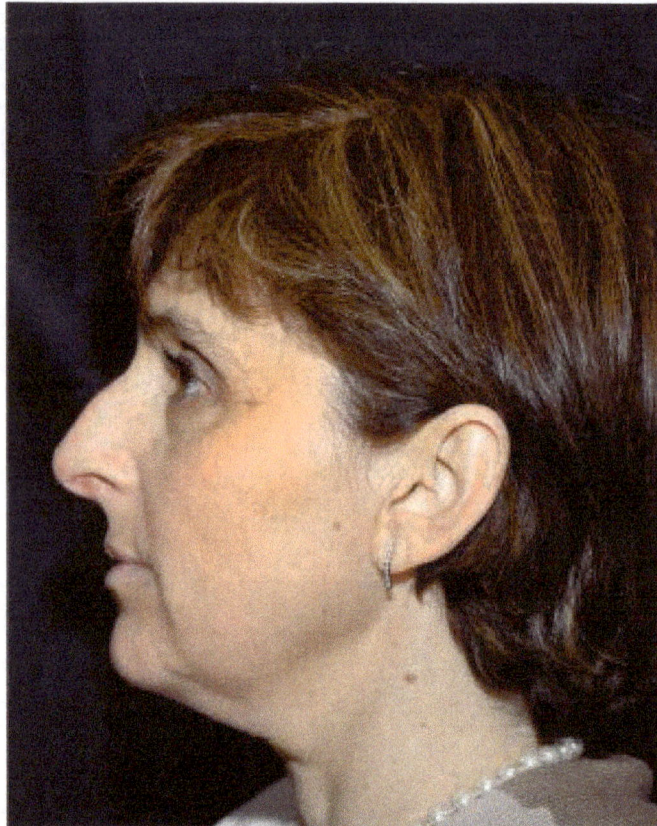

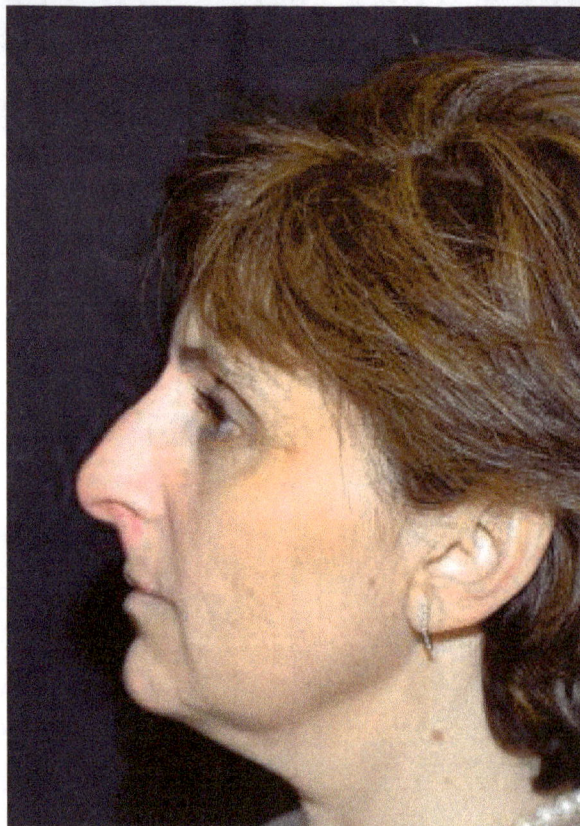

Figures 13-14. Rhinofiller pre-operative (upper) and post-operative (lower) immediate results, lateral view.

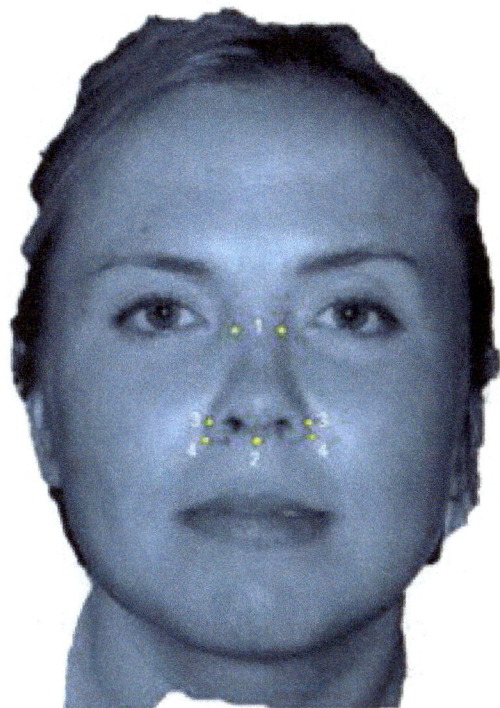

MUSCLE	ACTION	DOSE
1) Transverse Nasalis	Shortens Nose, Bunny lines	1-2 U per side
2) Depressor septi Nasi	Lowers tip, decrease projection	1-2 U
3) Dilator Naris	Dilates Narines, lowers tip	1-2U per side
4) Levator angulis oris alaeque nasi	Raises Upper lip, Gummy smile	5U per side

Figure 15. Summary of paranasal muscles and botulinum toxin doses.

Author details

Sebastian Torres[1*] and Tito Marianetti[2]

*Address all correspondence to: storres100@gmail.com

1 Plastic and Maxillofacial Surgery, Private Practice, Rome, Italy

2 Consultant in Maxillofacial Surgery, Private practice, Rome, Italy

References

[1] Rees TD. Aesthetic Plastic Surgery. Philadelphia, PA: WB Saunders; 1980.

[2] Paun SH, Nolst Trenité G. Revision rhinoplasty: an overview of deformities and techniques. Facial Plast Surg 2008; 24 (3):271–287.

[3] Adamson PA. The failed rhinoplasty. In: Current Therapy in Otolaringology Head and Neck Surgery. Toronto, ON: BC Decker; 1990: 137–44.

[4] Romo TIII, Sonne J, Choe KS, Sclafani AP. Revision rhinoplasty. Facial Plast Surg 2003; 19: 299–307.

[5] Rod J. Rohrich, William P. Adams, Jamil Ahmad, Jack Gunter. Dallas Rhinoplasty: Nasal Surgery by the Masters, Third Edition. Dallas, TX , USA; 2014. CRC Press.

[6] Sheen JH. Spreader graft: a method of reconstructing the roof of the middle nasal vault following rhinoplasty. Facial Plast Surg 1984; 73: 230–239.

[7] Boccieri A, Pascali M. Septal crossbar graft for the correction of the crooked nose. Plast Reconstr Surg 2003; 11: 629–638.

[8] Toriumi DM. Structure approach in rhinoplasty. Facial Plast Surg Clin North Am 2005; 13: 93–113.

[9] Sheen JH. Secondary rhinoplasty. Plast Reconstr Surg 1975; 56 (2): 137–145.

[10] Kridel RW. Septal perforation repair. Otolaryngol Clin North Am 1999; 32 (4): 695–724.

[11] Castelnuovo P, Ferreli F, Khodaei I, Palma P. Anterior ethmoidal artery septal flap for the management of septal perforation. Arch Facial Plast Surge 2011; 13 (6): 411–414.

[12] Toriumi DM, Josen J, Weinberger M, Tardy ME Jr. Use of alar batten grafts for correction of nasal valve collapse. Arch Otolaryngol Head Neck Surg 1997; 123: 802–808.

[13] Kridel RW, Soliemanzadeh P. Tip grafts in revision rhinoplasty. Facial Plast Surg Clin North Am 2006; 14: 331–341.

[14] Peck GC. The onlay graft for nasal tip projection. Plast Reconstr Surg 1983; 71 (1): 27–39.

[15] Peer LA. Cartilage grafting. Br J Plast Surg 1954; 7(3): 250–262.

[16] Boccieri A. Subtotal reconstruction of the nasal septum using a conchal reshaped graft. Ann Plast Surg 2004; 53(2): 118–125.

[17] Boccieri A, Macro C. Septal considerations in revision rhinoplasty. Facial Plast Surg Clin North Am 2006; 14: 357–371.

[18] Soliemanzadeh P, Kridel RW. Nasal tip overprojection: algorithm of surgical deprojection techniques and introduction of medial crural overlay. Arch Facial Plast Surg 2005; 7(6): 374–380.

[19] Kridel RWH. Dome truncation for management of the overproyected nasal tip. Ann Plast Surg 1990; 24 (5):385–396.

[20] Kridel RW, Chiu RJ. The management of alar columellar disproportion in revision rhinoplasty. Facial Plast Surg Clin North Am 2006; 14: 313–329.

[21] Fomon S, Bell JW, Berger EL, Goldman IB, Neivert H, Schattner A. New approach to ventral deflections of the nasal septum. AMA Arch Otolaryngol 1951; 54 (4): 357–366.

[22] Braccini F, Dohan Ehrenfest DM. [Medical rhinoplasty: rational for atraumatic nasal modelling using botulinum toxin and fillers]. Rev Laryongol Oto Rhinol (Bord). 2008;129(4–5):233–238.

[23] Kurkjian TJ et al. Soft-tissue fillers in rhinoplasty. Plast Reconstr Surg. 2014;133(2):121e–126e. 3.

[24] Wang YF et al. A woman's secret. Filler rhinoplasty with Radiesse (Merz Aesthetics, San Mateo, CA) and gold thread implantation. Ann Emerg Med. 2013;62(3):224, 234.

[25] Jasin ME. Nonsurgical rhinoplasty using dermal fillers. Facial Plast Surg Clin North Am. 2013;21(2):241–252.

[26] Humphrey CD et al. Soft tissue fillers in the nose. Aesthet Surg J. 2009;29(6): 477–484.

[27] Rivkin A. A prospective study of non-surgical primary rhinoplasty using a polymethylmethacrylate injectable implant. Dermatol Surg. 2014;40(3): 305–313.

[28] Kim YS et al. The anatomical origin and course of the angular artery regarding its clinical implications. Dermatol Surg. 2014;40(10):1070–1076.

[29] Saban Y et al. Nasal arterial vasculature: medical and surgical applications. Arch Facial Plast Surg. 2012;14(6):429–436.

[30] Lee HJ et al. Description of a novel anatomic venous structure in the nasoglabellar area. J Craniofac Surg. 2014;25(2):633–635.

[31] Hanke CW et al. Abscess formation and local necrosis after treatment with Zyderm or Zyplast collagen implant. J Am Acad Dermatol. 1991;25:319.

[32] Manafi A et al. Nasal alar necrosis following hyaluronic acid injection into nasolabial folds: a case report. World J Plast Surg. 2015;4(1):74–78.

[33] Chou CC et al. Choroid vascular occlusion and ischemic optic neuropathy after facial calcium hydroxyapatite injection- a case report. BMC Surg. 2015;15:21.

[34] Chen Y et al. Fundus artery occlusion caused by cosmetic facial injections. Chin Med J (Engl). 2014;127(8):1434–1437.

[35] Kim SN et al. Panophthalmoplegia and vision loss after cosmetic nasal dorsum injection. J Clin Neurosci. 2014;21(4): 678–680.

[36] Honart JF et al. A case of nasal tip necrosis after hyaluronic acid injection. Ann Chir Plast Esthet. 2013;58(6):676–679.

[37] Tracy L et al. Calcium hydroxylapatite associated soft tissue necrosis: a case report and treatment guidelines. J Plast Reconstr Aesthet Surg. 2014;67(4):564–568.

[38] Kim YJ, Choi KS. Bilateral blindness after filler injection. Plast Reconstr Surg. 2013;131(2):298e–299e.

[39] Park SW et al. Iatrogenic retinal artery occlusion caused by cosmetic facial filler injections. Am J Ophthalmol. 2012;154(4):653–662.e1.

[40] Sung MS et al. Ocular ischemia and ischemic oculomotor nerve palsy after vascular embolization of injectable calcium hydroxylapatite filler. Ophthal Plast Reconstr Surg. 2010;26(4):289–291.

[41] Beleznay K et al. Vascular compromise from soft tissue augmentation: experience with 12 cases and recommendations for optimal outcomes. J Clin Aesthet Dermatol. 2014;7(9):37–43.

[42] Kim SG et al. Salvage of nasal skin in a case of venous compromise after hyaluronic acid filler injection using prostaglandin E. Dermatol Surg. 2011;37(12):1817–1879.

[43] Menick FJ. Practical details of nasal reconstruction. Plast Reconstr Surg. 2013;131(4): 613e–630e.

[44] Menick FJ. Aesthetic and reconstructive rhinoplasty: a continuum. J Plast Reconstr Aesthet Surg. 2012;65(9):1169–1174.

[45] Sung HM et al. Case reports of adipose-derived stem cell therapy for nasal skin necrosis after filler injection. Arch Plast Surg. 2012;39(1):51–54

Permissions

All chapters in this book were first published in ATAOMS, by InTech Open; hereby published with permission under the Creative Commons Attribution License or equivalent. Every chapter published in this book has been scrutinized by our experts. Their significance has been extensively debated. The topics covered herein carry significant findings which will fuel the growth of the discipline. They may even be implemented as practical applications or may be referred to as a beginning point for another development.

The contributors of this book come from diverse backgrounds, making this book a truly international effort. This book will bring forth new frontiers with its revolutionizing research information and detailed analysis of the nascent developments around the world.

We would like to thank all the contributing authors for lending their expertise to make the book truly unique. They have played a crucial role in the development of this book. Without their invaluable contributions this book wouldn't have been possible. They have made vital efforts to compile up to date information on the varied aspects of this subject to make this book a valuable addition to the collection of many professionals and students.

This book was conceptualized with the vision of imparting up-to-date information and advanced data in this field. To ensure the same, a matchless editorial board was set up. Every individual on the board went through rigorous rounds of assessment to prove their worth. After which they invested a large part of their time researching and compiling the most relevant data for our readers.

The editorial board has been involved in producing this book since its inception. They have spent rigorous hours researching and exploring the diverse topics which have resulted in the successful publishing of this book. They have passed on their knowledge of decades through this book. To expedite this challenging task, the publisher supported the team at every step. A small team of assistant editors was also appointed to further simplify the editing procedure and attain best results for the readers.

Apart from the editorial board, the designing team has also invested a significant amount of their time in understanding the subject and creating the most relevant covers. They scrutinized every image to scout for the most suitable representation of the subject and create an appropriate cover for the book.

The publishing team has been an ardent support to the editorial, designing and production team. Their endless efforts to recruit the best for this project, has resulted in the accomplishment of this book. They are a veteran in the field of academics and their pool of knowledge is as vast as their experience in printing. Their expertise and guidance has proved useful at every step. Their uncompromising quality standards have made this book an exceptional effort. Their encouragement from time to time has been an inspiration for everyone.

The publisher and the editorial board hope that this book will prove to be a valuable piece of knowledge for researchers, students, practitioners and scholars across the globe.

List of Contributors

Fatih Özan
Faculty of Dentistry, Department of Oral and Maxillofacial Surgery, AbantİzzetBaysal University, Bolu, Turkey

Metin Şençimen and Aydın Gülses
Department of Dental Sciences, Department of Oral and Maxillofacial Surgery, Gülhane Military Medical Academy, Ankara, Turkey

Mustafa Ayna
Center for Implant Dentistry, Duisburg, Germany

Jamilian Abdolreza
Department of Orthodontics, Islamic Azad University, Tehran Dental Branch, Cranio Maxillofacial Research Centre, Tehran, Iran

Khosravi Saeed
Tehran University of Medical Sciences, Tehran, Iran

Darnahal Alireza
Tehran Dental Branch, Islamic Azad University, Tehran, Iran

Ruggero Rodriguez y Baena, Silvana Rizzo, Antonio Graziano and Saturnino Marco Lupi
Department of Clinico Surgical, Diagnostic and Pediatric Sciences, School of Dentistry,University of Pavia, Pavia, Italy

Farzin Sarkarat and Rouzbeh Kahali
Department of Oral and Maxillofacial Surgery, CMF Research Center, Buali Hospital, Islamic Azad University of Medical Sciences, Tehran, Iran

Farshid Kavandi
Department of Oral and Maxillofacial Surgery, Shahid Beheshti University of Medical Sciences, Tehran, Iran

Mohammad Hosein Kalantar Motamedi
Trauma Research Center, Baqiyatallah University of Medical Science and Islamic Azad University of Medical Sciences, Tehran, Iran

Seied Omid Keyhan
Department of Oral and Maxillofacial Surgery, Shahid Sadoughi & Shahid Beheshti University of Medical Sciences, Dental Research Center, Yazd-Tehran, Iran

Sina Ghanean and Alireza Navabazam
Department of Oral and Maxillofacial Surgery, Shahid Sadoughi University of Medical Sciences, Yazd, Iran

Arash Khojasteh
Department of Oral and Maxillofacial Surgery, Shahid Beheshti University of Medical Sciences, Tehran, Iran. Dean, School of Advanced Technologies in Medicine, Tehran, Iran

Mohammad Hosein Amirzade Iranaq
Student Research Committee, Shahid Sadoughi University of Medical Sciences, Yazd, Iran

Jeffrey A. Elo
Division of Oral and Maxillofacial Surgery, Western University of Health Sciences College of Dental Medicine, Pomona, California, USA
Department of Oral and Maxillofacial Surgery, Loma Linda University Medical Center, Loma Linda, California, USA

Ho-Hyun Sun
Western University of Health Sciences College of Dental Medicine, Pomona, California, USA

Shahram Nazerani
Rasool Akram General Hospital, Iran Medical University of Medical Sciences, Tehran, Iran

Tina Nazerani
General Practitioner, Graz, Austria

Reza Tabrizi and Hassan Mir Mohammad Sadeghi
Department of Oral and Maxillofacial Surgery, Shahid Beheshti University of Medical Sciences, Tehran, Iran

Sebastian Torres
Plastic and Maxillofacial Surgery, Private Practice, Rome, Italy

Tito Marianetti
Consultant in Maxillofacial Surgery, Private practice, Rome, Italy

Index